Donated by
Sensodyne.
(GlaxoSmithKline)

70

Dental Erosion

Monographs in Oral Science

Vol. 20

Series Editor

G.M. Whitford   *Augusta, Ga.*

KARGER

....

Dental Erosion

From Diagnosis to Therapy

Volume Editor

Adrian Lussi   Bern

52 figures, 37 in color, and 22 tables, 2006

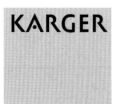

KARGER

Basel · Freiburg · Paris · London · New York ·
Bangalore · Bangkok · Singapore · Tokyo · Sydney

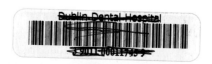

· ·

Adrian Lussi
Department of Preventive, Restorative and Pediatric Dentistry
School of Dental Medicine
University of Bern
Freiburgstrasse 7
CH–3010 Bern (Switzerland)

Library of Congress Cataloging-in-Publication Data

Dental erosion : from diagnosis to therapy / volume editor, Adrian Lussi.
      p. ; cm. – (Monographs in oral science, ISSN 0077-0892 ; v. 20)
   Includes bibliographical references and index.
   ISBN 3-8055-8097-5 (hard cover : alk. paper)
   1. Teeth–Erosion.   I. Lussi, Adrian. II. Series.
   [DNLM: 1. Tooth Erosion.   W1 MO568E v.20 2006 / WU 140
   D4135 2006]
   RK340.D46 2006
   617.6'3–dc22

2006008087

Bibliographic Indices. This publication is listed in bibliographic services, including Current Contents® and Index Medicus.

© Copyright 2006 by S. Karger AG, P.O. Box, CH–4009 Basel (Switzerland)
www.karger.com
Printed in Switzerland on acid-free paper by Reinhardt Druck, Basel
ISSN 0077–0892
ISBN 3–8055–8097–5

Contents

....
List of Contributors

Martin Addy, Prof. Dr.
Restorative Dentistry (Perio)
University of Bristol Dental Hospital
and School
Lower Maudlin Street
Bristol BS1 2LY (United Kingdom)
E-Mail Martin.Addy@bristol.ac.uk

Birgit Angmar-Månsson, Prof. Dr.
Department of Cariology and
Endodontology, Institute of Odontology
Karolinska Institutet, Huddinge
Alfred Nobels Alle 8, Box 4064
S–14104 Huddinge (Sweden)
Fax +46 8 711 83 43
E-Mail Birgit.Angmar-Mansson@ki.se

Thomas Attin, Prof. Dr.
University of Zurich
Center for Dental and Oral Medicine and
Maxillo-facial Surgery
Clinic for Preventive Dentistry
Periodontology and Cariology
Plattenstrasse 11
CH–8032 Zürich
Fax +41 44 634 43 08

David Bartlett, Dr.
Department of Prosthodontics, GKT
Dental Institute
Floor 25, Guy's Tower, St. Thomas' Street
London Bridge, London SE1 9RT
(United Kingdom)
Fax +44 020 71881792
E-Mail david.bartlett@kcl.ac.uk

John Featherstone, Prof. Dr.
Department of Preventive and Restorative
Dental Sciences
University of California at San Francisco
Room 0603, Box 0758
707 Parnassus Avenue, San Francisco
CA 94143 (USA), Fax +1 415 476 0926
E-Mail jdbf@ucsf.edu

Carolina Ganss, PD Dr.
Department of Conservative and Preventive
Dentistry, Dental Clinic
Justus Liebig University Giessen
Schlangenzahl 14
DE–35392 Giessen (Germany)
Fax +49 641 99 46 169
E-Mail Carolina.Ganss@dentist.med.
uni-giessen.de

Anne Grüninger, Dr.
Department of Preventive, Restorative and
Pediatric Dentistry
School of Dental Medicine
University of Bern
Freiburgstrasse 7
CH–3010 Bern (Switzerland)
Fax +41 31 632 98 75
E-Mail amvv@bluewin.ch

Anderson T. Hara, Dr.
Department of Preventive and Community
Dentistry, Indiana University
School of Dentistry
415 N. Lansing Street
Indianapolis, IN 46202-2876 (USA)
Fax +1 317 274 54 25
E-Mail ahara@iupui.edu

Elmar Hellwig, Prof. Dr.
Department of Operative Dentistry and
Periodontology
University Clinic of Dentistry, Freiburg
Hugstetter Strasse 55
DE–79106 Freiburg (Germany)
Fax +49 761 270 47 62
E-Mail hellwig@zmk2.ukl.uni-freiburg.de

Thomas Jaeggi, Dr.
Department of Preventive, Restorative and
Pediatric Dentistry
School of Dental Medicine
University of Bern
Freiburgstrasse 7
CH–3010 Bern (Switzerland)
Fax +41 31 632 98 75
E-Mail thom.jaeggi@bluewin.ch

Adrian Lussi, Prof. Dr.
Department of Preventive, Restorative and
Pediatric Dentistry
School of Dental Medicine
University of Bern
Freiburgstrasse 7
CH–3010 Bern (Switzerland)
Fax +41 31 632 98 75
E-Mail adrian.lussi@zmk.unibe.ch

Peter Shellis, Dr.
Restorative Dentistry (Perio)
University of Bristol Dental Hospital
and School
Lower Maudlin Street
Bristol BS1 2LY (United Kingdom)
E-Mail R.P.Shellis@bristol.ac.uk

Nicola West, Dr.
Restorative Dentistry (Perio)
University of Bristol Dental Hospital
and School
Lower Maudlin Street
Bristol BS1 2LY (United Kingdom)
E-Mail N.X.West@bristol.ac.uk

Dominick Zero, Prof. Dr.
Department of Preventive and Community
Dentistry, Indiana University
School of Dentistry
415 N. Lansing Street
Indianapolis, IN 46202-2876 (USA)
Fax +1 317 274 54 25
E-Mail dzero@iupui.edu

Acknowledgments

This book, which is the first of its kind to deal with all aspects of erosive tooth wear, was generously sponsored by the following bodies:

GlaxoSmithKline
Procter&Gamble
Curaden
Gaba
Clincial Research Foundation

Sincere thanks goes to the experts who reviewed all chapters. Their commitments have ensured a high standard of the book.

Foreword

Dental Erosion: A challenge for the 21st century! This monograph offers a guide towards better oral health in the future. Erosive tooth wear is a multifactorial condition of growing concern to the clinician and the subject of extensive research – a view supported by the literature and impressions from many international conferences over recent decades. However, until now, no attempt has been made to collect and organize the available information in a single book. This volume of *Monographs in Oral Science* is the first book dealing solely with erosive tooth wear.

The thirteen chapters of the book present a broad spectrum of views on dental erosion, from the molecular level to behavioral aspects and trends in society. The multifactorial etiological pattern of erosive tooth wear is emphasized and is a strand connecting the different chapters of the book. It starts with the definition of erosion and describes the interaction of attrition, abrasion and erosion in tooth wear. The chapters on diagnosis of erosion, and prevalence, incidence and distribution of the condition are followed by a chapter on the chemistry of erosion. Under the heading extrinsic causes of erosion, several factors are analyzed and illustrated, amongst which are the consequences of our changing life styles and the effects of oral hygiene products and acidic medicines. The chapter on intrinsic causes of erosion focuses on gastroesophageal reflux disease and related issues. A separate chapter is devoted to dental erosion in children. Methods of assessment of dental erosion are presented and critically evaluated, concluding that the complex nature of erosive mineral loss and dissolution might not readily be encompassed by a single technique: a more comprehensive approach combining several different methods is recommended. The last three chapters cover dentinal hypersensitivity, risk assessment and preventive measures, and, finally, restorative options for erosive lesions.

Each chapter has a comprehensive list of references, encouraging the reader to consult the original articles for more details. Instructive intraoral photographs illustrate the text and guide the reader. An unusual step is that every chapter was reviewed not only by the editor, but also by two external reviewers, ensuring the highest of standards.

This monograph describes current concepts of dental erosion and presents an overview of the literature, with special reference to clinically relevant implications. It is not only suitable for faculty members and researchers, but may also be recommended for dental students, practitioners and other dental professionals who are committed to preventing and treating dental erosion.

Birgit Angmar-Månsson, Stockholm

Lussi A (ed): Dental Erosion.
Monogr Oral Sci. Basel, Karger, 2006, vol 20, pp 1–8

....

Erosive Tooth Wear – A Multifactorial Condition of Growing Concern and Increasing Knowledge

A. Lussi

Department of Preventive, Restorative and Pediatric Dentistry, School of Dental Medicine, University of Bern, Bern, Switzerland

Abstract

Dental erosion is often described solely as a surface phenomenon, unlike caries where it has been established that the destructive effects involve both the surface and the subsurface region. However, besides removal and softening of the surface, erosion may show dissolution of mineral underneath the surface. There is some evidence that the presence of this condition is growing steadily. Hence, erosive tooth wear is becoming increasingly significant in the management of the long-term health of the dentition. What is considered as an acceptable amount of wear is dependent on the anticipated lifespan of the dentition and, therefore, is different for deciduous compared to permanent teeth. However, erosive damage to the permanent teeth occurring in childhood may compromise the growing child's dentition for their entire lifetime and may require repeated and increasingly complex and expensive restoration. Therefore, it is important that diagnosis of the tooth wear process in children and adults is made early and adequate preventive measures are undertaken. These measures can only be initiated when the risk factors are known and interactions between them are present. A scheme is proposed which allows the possible risk factors and their relation to each other to be examined.

Change of Perception

Erosive tooth wear has for many years been a condition of little interest to clinical dental practice or dental public health. Diagnosis was seldom made, especially in the early stages, and there was little if anything that could be done to intervene in the early stages. However, perceptions are now changing. In the year 1995, a special issue of the *European Journal of Oral Science* entitled 'Etiology, mechanisms and implications of dental erosions' was published [1]. It was stated in the preface that dental erosion is an area of research and clinical practice that will undoubtedly experience expansion in the next decade. Indeed, in the last decade erosion has attracted a great amount of research, with subsequent progression in the field. Whilst in the 1970s less than 5 studies per year were published about erosion, this number was still below 10 in the 1980s and has nowadays increased to about 50 studies per year. (Erosive) tooth wear is becoming increasingly significant in the long term health of the dentition and the overall well-being of those who suffer its effects. Following the decline in tooth loss in the 20th century, the increasing longevity of teeth in the 21st century will render the clinically deleterious effect of wear more demanding upon the preventive and restorative skills of the dental professional [2]. Awareness of dental erosion by the public is still not widespread, and dental professionals worldwide are sometimes confused by its signs and symptoms, and its similarities and differences from the other categories of tooth wear namely abrasion, attrition and abfraction. In its early stages, and for the vast majority of the population, the changes seen in tooth erosion are of only cosmetic significance. In a survey in England, 34% of the children were aware of tooth erosion but only 8% could recall their dentist mentioning the condition [3]. Forty percent of children believed incorrectly that the best way to avoid erosion was regular toothbrushing which shows some lack of information or misunderstanding. In addition, the awareness of dentists was considered low [3].

Change of Consumption of Acidic Foods and Beverages

As lifestyles have changed through the decades, the total amount and frequency of consumption of acidic foods and drinks have also changed. Soft drink consumption in the USA increased by 300% in 20 years, [4] and serving sizes increased from 185 g (6.6 oz) in the 1950s to 340 g (12 oz) in the 1960s and to 570 g (20 oz) in the late 1990s. Around the year 1995, between 56 and 85% of children at school in the USA consumed at least one soft drink daily with the highest amounts ingested by adolescent males. Of this group, 20% consumed four or more servings daily [5]. Studies in children and adults have shown that this number of servings per day is associated with the presence and progression of erosion when other risk factors are present [6, 7].

It becomes obvious that with the increased popularity of soft drinks the consumption of milk may decrease in children and adolescents, which could result in calcium deficiency, thus jeopardizing the accrual of maximal peak bone mass at a critical time in life [8].

Change of Prevalence of Erosion

National dental surveys are not routinely undertaken and when conducted seldom have included measures of tooth wear, specifically erosion. Erosion was first included in the UK childrens' dental health survey in 1993 and is repeated periodically. The prevalence of erosion was seen to have increased from the time of the children's dental health survey in 1993 to the study of 4- to 18-year-olds in 1996/1997 [9]. There was a trend towards a higher prevalence of erosion in children aged between 3 1/2 and 4 1/2 years, and in those who consumed carbonated drinks on most days, compared with toddlers consuming these drinks less often. In another UK study, 1,308 children were examined at the age of 12 years and 2 years later. Five percent of the subjects aged 12 years and 13% 2 years later had deep enamel lesions. Dentinal lesions were found in 2% of the examined subjects at the age of 12 years and rose to 9% 2 years later. The incidence of new cases also increased. Twelve percent of 12-year-old children who demonstrated no evidence of erosion developed the condition over the subsequent 2 years. New and more advanced lesions were seen in 27% of the children over the study period [10]. Active erosive lesions will progress when no adequate preventive measures are implemented (figs. 1–3). To determine the progression of erosive defects 55 persons were examined twice on two occasions six years apart [7]. All persons were informed about the risk of erosive tooth wear but no active preventive care during the study period was performed. A distinct progression of erosion on occlusal and facial surfaces was found. The occurrence of occlusal erosions with involvement of dentine rose from 3 to 8% (26–30-years-old at the first examination) and from 8 to 26% (46–50-years-old at the first examination). The increase in facial erosions was smaller but again more marked for the older group. In this longitudinal study, the subjective evaluation of dentine hypersensitivity remained unchanged despite the marked increase of erosive and wedge-shaped defects. Dentine hypersensitivity is a relatively common phenomenon and tooth wear, specifically erosion, has been implicated as a predisposing factor [11]. However, no conclusive data are available which would show an increase of dentine hypersensitivity with increasing acidic consumption or erosive tooth wear. Clearly, more research is needed in this field.

Early Diagnosis

Early diagnosis is important. Dental professionals will typically ignore or overlook the very early stages dismissing minor tooth surface loss as a normal and inevitable occurrence of daily living, being 'within normal limits' and thus not appropriate for any specific interventive activity. Only at the later stages in

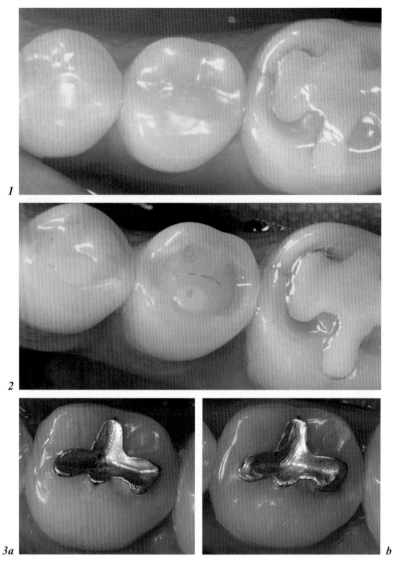

Fig. 1. Occlusal erosive tooth wear with involvement of dentine with a composite filling rising above the level of the adjacent tooth surface. Age of the patient: 30 years. Known risk factors: soft drinks (sip-wise), gastroesophageal reflux.

Fig. 2. Same patient as in figure 1 (5 years later). The progression on the premolars and on the first molar is clearly visible.

Fig. 3. *a* Occlusal erosive tooth wear of a child aged 14 years. He suffered from dentine hypersensitivity. Known risk factors: gastroesophageal reflux, ice tea, acidic beverages. *b* Same patient 2 1/2 years later. Progression is clearly visible.

which dentine has become exposed and possibly sensitive, and the appearance and shape of the teeth altered that the condition becomes evident at routine examination. There is no device available for the specific detection of dental erosion in routine practice. Therefore, the clinical appearance is the most important feature for dental professionals to diagnose dental erosion. This is of particular importance in the early stage of erosive tooth wear. The appearance of a smooth silky-glazed appearance, intact enamel along the gingival margin, change in color and cupping and grooving on occlusal surfaces are some typical signs of early erosion. However, it is difficult to diagnose erosion at an early stage and it can be very difficult to determine if dentine is exposed or not [12]. Even if a clinician is able to diagnose tooth wear, the differential diagnosis of erosion, abrasion or attrition may be a challenge either through lack of awareness of the multifactorial and overlying etiologies. It is possible to use disclosing agents to render dentine involvement visible. Only a dentist with the diagnostic capability of distinguishing early erosion from the other noncarious defects will be in a position to deliver timely preventive measures. Indeed, these conditions may occur simultaneously. In children, the most commonly reported areas with wear are occlusal surfaces of molars (fig. 3) and incisal surfaces of incisors. These surfaces are also associated with attrition and it can be difficult to separate what is being caused by erosion from what is being caused by other tooth wear factors [13]. For these and other reasons the terms 'erosion' and 'erosive tooth wear' are used in this book interchangeably demonstrating the overlapping nature of this condition.

Change of Knowledge and Risk Factors

Erosion is often described solely as a surface phenomenon, unlike caries where it has been established that the destructive effects are both on the surface and within the subsurface region. However, the pathophysiology of erosion is more complex. When a solution comes in contact, with enamel, it has to diffuse first through the acquired pellicle and only thereafter can it interact with enamel [see chapter 6 by Featherstone et al., this vol, pp 66–76]. The acquired pellicle is a biofilm, free of bacteria, covering oral hard and soft tissues. It is composed of mucins, glycoproteins and proteins, amongst which are several enzymes [14]. On the surface of enamel, the acid with its hydrogen ion (or a chelating agent) will start to dissolve the enamel crystal. First, the prism sheath area and then the prism core are dissolved, leaving the well-known honeycomb appearance [15]. Fresh, unionized acid will then eventually diffuse [16] into the interprismatic areas of enamel and dissolve further mineral underneath the surface, in the sub-surface region [17, 18]. This will lead to an outflow of ions and subsequently to a local pH rise in the tooth substance and in the liquid surface

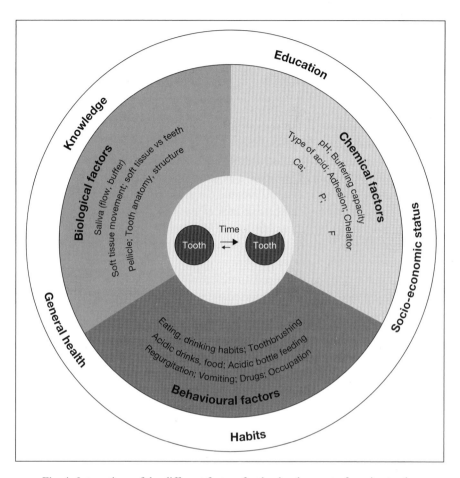

Fig. 4. Interactions of the different factors for the development of erosive tooth wear.

layer in close proximity to the enamel surface [18]. The events in dentine are in principle the same but are even more complex. Due to the high content of organic material, diffusion of the demineralizing agent (i.e. acid) deeper into the region and the outward flux of tooth mineral are hindered by the organic dentine matrix [19]. It has been assumed that the organic dentine matrix has a sufficient buffering capacity to retard further demineralization and that chemical or mechanical degradation of the dentine matrix promotes demineralization [20, 21].

These erosive processes are halted when no new acids and/or chelating substances are provided. An increase in agitation (e.g. when a drink is swished around the mouth) will enhance the dissolution process because the solution on the surface layer adjacent to enamel will be readily renewed [22]. Further, the amount of drink in the mouth in relation to the amount and flow of saliva present will modify the process of dissolution [2]. There are many more factors which are involved in and interact with erosive tooth wear. Figure 4 is an attempt to reveal the multifactorial predisposing factors and etiologies of the erosive condition, which seems to be steadily rising in western societies. Many biological, behavioral and chemical factors are interacting with the tooth surface, which over time, may either wear it away, or indeed protect it depending upon their fine balance (see chapter 7 by Lussi et al., this vol, pp 77–118 and chapter 8 by Bartlett, this vol, pp 119–139). Hydrogen ion concentration (pH) alone does not explain erosive potential of a foodstuff; titratable acidity, calcium, phosphate, fluoride levels and other factors must also be considered. The interplay of all these factors (fig. 4) is crucial and helps explain why some individuals exhibit more erosion than others, even if they are exposed to exactly the same acid challenge in their diets. In the initial stage a certain degree of repair should be possible as there is a subsurface component of the process which is symbolized with the short (back reaction) arrow in figure 4. As known in the carious process [23] the factors listed in the outer circle will influence the whole process of erosion development or defense further. Comprehensive knowledge of the different risk and protective factors is a prerequisite to initiate adequate preventive measures. People who show signs and symptoms of erosion are often not aware of, and may easily be confused by, the erosive potential of some drinks and foodstuffs. Only when a comprehensive case history is undertaken will all the risk factors be revealed. However, a thorough knowledge of the erosive potential of drinks and foodstuffs is needed by the dentist, to determine the patient's risk and to bring it in to context with the behavioral and biological factors. Knowing these factors, the reported symptoms (thermal or tactile sensitivity) and signs evident on clinical examination, and putting them in relation to the wishes, hopes and possibilities of the individual patient enables the dentist to initiate adequate preventive (noninterventive) and therapeutic (interventive) measures. When a restoration becomes inevitable, in all situations, the preparations have to follow the principles of minimally invasive treatment. In no case may early diagnosis of erosive tooth wear be an excuse for a restoration. Instead preventive measures must be initiated to reduce the erosive challenge and to increase the protective and defensive factors thus bringing this equilibrium back to the oral environment.

References

1   Ten Cate JM, Imfeld T: Dental erosion (preface). Eur J Oral Sci 1996;104:149.
2   Zero T, Lussi A: Erosion – chemical and biological factors of importance to the dental practitioner. Int Dent J 2005;55:285–290.

3   Dugmore CR, Rock WP: Awareness of tooth erosion in 12 year old children and primary care dental practitioners. Community Dent Health 2003;20:223–227.

4   Calvadini C, Siega-Riz AM, Popkin BM: US adolescent food intake trends from 1965 to 1996. Arch Dis Child 2000;83:18–24.

5   Gleason P, Suitor C: Children's Diets in the Mid-1990s: Dietary intake and Its Relationship with School Meal Participation. Alexandria, US Department of Agriculture, Food and Nutrition Service, Office of Analysis, Nutrition and Evaluation, 2001.

6   O'Sullivan EA, Curzon MEJ: A comparison of acidic dietary factors in children with and without dental erosion. J Dent Child 2000;67:186–192.

7   Lussi A, Schaffner M: Progression of and risk factors for dental erosion and wedge-shaped defects over a 6-year period. Caries Res 2000;34:182–187.

8   American Academy of Pediatrics, Committee on School Health: Soft drinks in schools. Pediatrics 2004;113:152–153.

9   Nunn JH, Gordon PH, Morris AJ, Pine CM, Walker A: Dental erosion – changing prevalence? A review of British National childrens' surveys. Int J Paediatr Dent 2003;13:98–105.

10 Dugmore CR, Rock WP: The progression of tooth erosion in a cohort of adolescents of mixed ethnicity. Int J Paediatr Dent 2003;13:295–303.

11 Addy M: Tooth brushing, tooth wear and dentine hypersensitivity – are they associated? Int Dent J 2005;55:261–267.

12 Ganss C, Klimek J, Lussi A: Accuracy and consistency of the visual diagnosis of exposed dentine on worn occlusal/incisal surfaces. Caries Res, in press.

13 Bartlett D: The implication of laboratory research on tooth wear and erosion. Oral Dis 2005;11:3–6.

14 Hannig C, Hannig M, Attin T: Enzymes in the acquired enamel pellicle. Eur J Oral Sci 2005;113:2–13.

15 Meurman JH, Frank RM: Scanning electron microscopic study of the effect of salivary pellicle on enamel erosion. Caries Res 1991;25:1–6.

16 Featherstone JDB, Rodgers BE: Effect of acetic, lactic and other organic acids on the formation of artificial carious lesions. Caries Res 1981;15:377–385.

17 Eisenburger M, Hughes J, West NX, Shellis RP, Addy M: The use of ultrasonication to study remineralisation of eroded enamel. Caries Res 2001;35:61–66.

18 Lussi A, Hellwig E: Erosive potential of oral care products. Caries Res 2001;35:52–56.

19 Hara AT, Ando M, Cury JA, Serra MC, Gonzalez-Cabezas C, Zero DT: Influence of the organic matrix on root dentine erosion by citric acid. Caries Res 2005;39:134–138.

20 Ganss C, Klimek J, Starck C: Quantitative analysis of the impact of the organic matrix on the fluoride effect on erosion progression in human dentine using longitudinal microradiography. Arch Oral Biol 2004;49:931–935.

21 Kleter GA, Damen JJ, Everts V, Niehof J, Ten Cate JM: The influence of the organic matrix on demineralization of bovine root dentin in vitro. J Dent Res 1994;73:1523–1539.

22 Shellis RP, Finke M, Eisenburger M, Parker DM, Addy M: Relationship between enamel erosion and liquid flow rate. Eur J Oral Sci 2005;113:232–238.

23 Fejerskov O: Changing paradigms in concepts on dental caries: consequences for oral health care. Caries Res 2004;38:182–191.

Prof. Dr. Adrian Lussi
Department of Preventive, Restorative and Pediatric Dentistry
School of Dental Medicine
University of Bern, Freiburgstrasse 7
CH–3010 Bern (Switzerland)

Lussi A (ed): Dental Erosion.
Monogr Oral Sci. Basel, Karger, 2006, vol 20, pp 9–16

....

Definition of Erosion and Links to Tooth Wear

C. Ganss

Department of Conservative and Preventive Dentistry,
Dental Clinic, Justus Liebig University Giessen, Giessen, Germany

Abstract

Erosive tissue loss is part of the physiological wear of teeth. Clinical features are an initial loss of tooth shine or luster, followed by flattening of convex structures, and, with continuing acid exposure, concavities form on smooth surfaces, or grooving and cupping occur on incisal/occlusal surfaces. Dental erosion must be distinguished from other forms of wear, but can also contribute to general tissue loss by surface softening, thus enhancing physical wear processes. The determination of dental erosion as a condition or pathology is relatively easy in the case of pain or endodontic complications, but is ambiguous in terms of function or aesthetics. The impact of dental erosion on oral health is discussed. However, it can be concluded that in most cases dental erosion is best described as a condition, with the acid being of nonpathological origin.

Definition of Erosive Tissue Loss

During a lifetime, teeth are exposed to a number of physical and chemical insults, which to a various extent contribute to the wear and tear of dental hard tissues.

The variety of processes include the friction of exogenous material (e.g. during mastication, toothbrushing, holding tools) forced over tooth substances (abrasion), the effect of antagonistic teeth (attrition), the impact of tensile and compressive forces during tooth flexure (abfraction), and the chemical dissolution of tooth mineral (erosion) (table 1). All of these factors to a greater or lesser extent occur in the dentition, and wear results from the simultaneous and/or synergistic action of these processes (see chapter 3 by Addy et al., this vol,

Table 1. Terminology, definition and etiology of various types of physical and chemical tooth wear

Terminology	Definition and etiology
Abrasion	Physical wear as a result of mechanical processes involving foreign substances or objects (three body wear) Etiological factors are oral hygiene procedures (e.g. excessive brushing/flossing, effect of abrasives in toothpastes), habits (e.g. holding objects), or occupational exposure to abrasive particles The resulting morphology of defects can be diffuse or localized depending on the predominant impact Wedge-shaped defects are also attributed to abrasion A special form of abrasion is demastication, which means wear from chewing food Tissue loss is located on incisal and/or occlusal surfaces and depends on the abrasiveness of the individual diet
Attrition	Physical wear as a result of the action of antagonistic teeth with no foreign substances intervening (two body wear) Characteristic features are antagonistic plane facets with sharp margins
Abfraction	Physical wear as a result of tensile or shear stress in the cemento-enamel region provoking microfractures in enamel and dentine (fatigue wear) Wedge-shaped defects are also attributed to abfraction
Erosion	Chemical wear as a result of extrinsic or intrinsic acids or chelators acting on plaque-free tooth surfaces Characteristic clinical features of (tribo) chemical wear are loss of surface structure, melted appearance, cupping or grooving on occlusal/incisal surfaces, and shallow concavities coronal from the cemento-enamel junction

pp 17–31). The morphology and severity of defects may substantially vary depending on the predominant etiological factor (fig. 1).

Dental erosion can be defined as dissolution of tooth by acids when the surrounding aqueous phase is undersaturated with respect to tooth mineral [1]. When the acidic challenge is acting for long enough, a clinically visible defect occurs. On smooth surfaces, the original luster of the tooth dulls. Later, the convex areas flatten or shallow concavities become present which are mostly located coronal to the enamel–cementum junction. On occlusal surfaces, cusps become rounded or cupped and edges of restorations appear to rise above the level of the adjacent tooth surfaces. In severe cases, the whole tooth morphology disappears and the vertical crown height can be significantly reduced (for morphology of erosive wear, see chapter 4 by Ganss et al., this vol, pp 32–43).

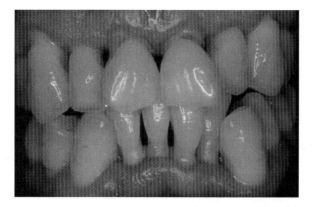

Fig. 1. Fifty-year-old woman with multiple forms of wear: 11 and 21 cervical abrasions due to abusive flossing, 13 and 23 wedge-shaped defects; 32–42 toothbrush abrasion.

The result of continuing acid exposure, however, is not only a clinically visible defect, but also a change in the physical properties of the remaining tooth surface. It is recognized that erosive demineralization results in a significant reduction in microhardness [2–4], making the softened surface more prone to mechanical impacts [5]. Although independent in origin, erosion is therefore linked to other forms of wear not only because it contributes to the individual overall rate of tooth tissue loss, but also by enhancing physical wear (see chapter 3 by Addy et al., this vol, pp 17–31).

Although listed in the International Classification of Diseases [6], erosive tissue loss cannot be regarded as pathology per se. Unlike caries and periodontitis, which should not occur at all, erosive and physical wear contribute to the physiological loss of tooth tissue occurring throughout life time.

Is Erosive Tooth Wear an Oral Disease?

Attempts have been made to distinguish between pathological and physiological loss of tooth tissues [7]:

'Tooth wear can be regarded as pathological if the teeth become so worn that they do not function effectively or seriously mar the appearance before they are lost for other causes or the patient dies. The distinction of acceptable and pathological wear at a given age is based upon the prediction of whether the tooth will survive the rate of wear'.

'Function' in a professional view means (1) the interplay of the dental arches (occlusion); (2) the action of musculature and temporo-mandibular joint, and (3) the biological integrity of teeth.

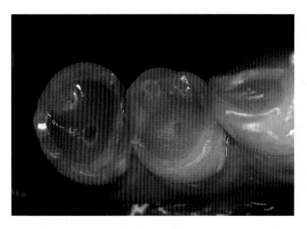

Fig. 2. Frank, and near pulp exposure (45 and 44) in a 58-year-old male with advanced wear of unknown etiology. He complained about a sudden pinprick-like feeling when chewing.

With continuing erosive demineralization and loss of enamel, formation of reactionary and reparative dentine and obturation of dentinal tubules are biologic responses that compensate for the loss of tissue. In the case that the progression of erosive wear exceeds the reparative capacity of the dentinal–pulp complex (fig. 2), and when excessive (erosive) wear occurs, possible complications are pain, pulpal inflammation, necrosis, and periapical pathology.

The prevalence of endodontic sequelae has not been systematically studied, but is estimated to occur in roughly 10% of patients with significant wear [8]. Pain, however, is not only induced by near or frank pulp exposure, but can occur as soon as dentine is exposed. The etiology of dentinal hypersensitivity has been extensively described, and it appears that the absence of a smear layer and patent tubules are the relevant factors, which would favor the exposure to acids as the primary etiology [9]. However, even if not studied systematically, hypersensitivity from the clinical experience appears as only a minor problem in most subjects with erosive wear.

Continuing hypersensitivity, acute pain or pulp necrosis with periapical inflammation would doubtlessly represent a pathological condition. However, even severe (erosive) tooth wear can be localized to single teeth or generalized without any clinical symptoms, a condition which refers to considerations regarding the significance of the morphology of teeth for occlusion, musculature, and joints.

The teeth of prehistoric hunter-gatherers are often characterized by extensive wear in both arches. Although a decrease in wear is seen on the dentition of

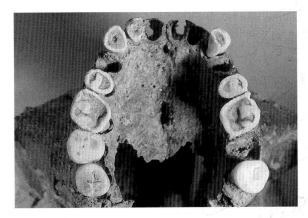

Fig. 3. Medieval subject (estimated age 50–70) with advanced generalized wear.

premodern and recent people, its presence appears to be a constant feature [10]. Observations from anthropologists therefore led to substantially different concepts of occlusion than those generally accepted in dentistry. Begg [11] suggested that an 'attritional occlusion' rather than a nonattritional occlusion is the anatomically and functionally correct feature. 'Attritional occlusion' refers to a dentition that is affected by various wear processes which are present in heavy-wear environments (fig. 3). Edge-to-edge occlusion and working/nonworking contacts are the major features in this concept, whereas scissors occlusion and interlocking cusp relation appear as a retention in a juvenile condition which is 'unexpected' if the history of the human body is considered. Since his publication, a number of aspects regarding this theory have been investigated, which are extensively reviewed by Kaifu et al. [12]. They considered tooth wear in the context of evolutionary adaptation and conclude: 'Our synthesis of the available evidence suggests that the human dentition is "designed" on the premise that extensive wear will occur'. In this concept, even extensive wear can be regarded as a condition rather than a pathology, provided that the amount of loss is related to the expected life span (for assessment of progression, see chapter 4 by Ganss et al., this vol, pp 32–43).

The concept of attritional occlusion is in stark contrast to theories generally accepted in dentistry. Most concepts of an ideal occlusion include a defined centric occlusion and a canine or group guidance without nonworking contacts. Probably, the most inflexible concept of an ideal nonattritional occlusion was presented by Lee [13]. He suggested that a physiological occlusion should feature a 4-mm overbite, 3-mm overjet, and on lateral excursions, canines cause the posterior teeth to disclude. But most importantly, he stated that teeth without any signs of wear were essential for a properly functioning dentition. The consequence of premise is that any wear of teeth, no matter how small, is regarded as pathological.

Based on the concept of a nonattritional occlusion, an enormous body of literature has been published regarding the role of occlusion in the etiology of temporo-mandibular disorders (TMD). Based on this concept, erosive tooth wear involving loss of occlusal morphology and resulting in a lack of canine or group guidance, nonworking contacts and loss of vertical height would increase the risk of developing TMD. However, clinical studies reveal none or weak associations between deviations from an ideal occlusion and TMD [14–17]. Correspondingly, there is no evidence that occlusal adjustment should be part of any recommended treatment for TMD [18]. Clinical studies investigating the association of TMD and generalized erosive tooth wear are absent, but several investigations on the morphology of the temporo-mandibular joint in prehistoric subjects with wear have been published. It has been demonstrated that struc-tural changes to the fossa and condyle occur either as degenerative (i.e. bony erosion, proliferation, or eburnation) [19, 20] or adaptive changes [21–23]. These studies, however, have obvious limitations at least as they cannot be cor-related with the clinical situation.

The professionals' description of function might significantly differ from a patient's perspective and, accordingly, clinical judgments have only limited power in interpreting oral health [24]. Considering the emotional and social significance of food, the individuals' need for function of the dentition would address mastica-tory ability, which comprises chewing capacity and chewing with comfort rather than the objective chewing efficiency. The finding that shortened dental arches with all molars missing was sufficient to satisfy most individual's needs [24], means the general relevance of wear for the masticatory ability is difficult to assess. Aesthetics, however, appears to be more important for many people than function [24]. Beauty has been closely associated with truth and goodness. Individuals endowed with physical beauty are seen as virtuous and trustful, and are given more social credit than subjects afflicted with ugliness. White teeth rep-resent health and youth, vice versa a worn and yellowish dentition is attributed to old age and loss of power. This notion is strongly supported by Rufenacht [25]. Even if it is assumed that there must be universal norms of aesthetics, beauty ideals are the result of culture and related to time and fashion. Hence, the con-cepts and impacts of bodily beauty vary considerably between people [26]. It is often the individual who first recognizes his or her tooth wear as a pathological condition. But it is the dentist's responsibility to consider the complexity sur-rounding the concepts of beauty and the sequelae of bodily changes, and, most importantly, to enhance the patients in making an informed decision particularly if extensive and expensive restorations are considered.

Considering the various aspects addressed above, it appears that the difference between a condition and pathology is dependent on the concepts of health and disease. Erosion might be considered to be pathological when occurring in combination with pain or acute endodontic complications. It is also reasonable to consider that minor to moderate tissue loss is a normal feature of the aging dentition. But in asymptomatic advanced erosive wear the differentiation between a physiological and pathological state becomes more difficult to distinguish. The question whether, and in which cases, erosion is an oral disease is currently open for debate. In general terms, though, dental erosion is best described as a condition brought upon by an acid insult, with the acid being of nonpathological origin.

Future research and discussion of the role of erosive tooth wear in oral health is needed, but the matter also appears to be stimulating for reflecting on concepts of health and disease in dentistry in general.

References

1   Larsen MJ: Chemical events during tooth dissolution. J Dent Res 1990;69(spec No):575–580.
2   Lussi A, Jaeggi T, Jaeggi-Schärer S: Prediction of the erosive potential of some beverages. Caries Res 1995;29:349–354.
3   Lussi A, Portmann P, Burhop B: Erosion on abraded dental hard tissues by acid lozenges: an in situ study. Clin Oral Invest 1997;1:191–194.
4   Maupome G, Diez-de-Bonilla J, Torres-Villasenor G, Andrade-Delgado LC, Castano VM: In vitro quantitative assessment of enamel microhardness after exposure to eroding immersion in a cola drink. Caries Res 1998;32:148–153.
5   Attin T, Koidl U, Buchalla W, Schaller HG, Kielbassa AM, Hellwig E: Correlation of microhardness and wear in differently eroded bovine dental enamel. Arch Oral Biol 1997;42: 243–250.
6   World Health Organisation: ICD-10 Online Version. International Statistical Classification of Diseases and Related Health Problems, 2003.
7   Smith BG, Knight JK: An index for measuring the wear of teeth. Br Dent J 1984;156:435–438.
8   Sivasithamparam K, Harbrow D, Vinczer E, Young WG: Endodontic sequelae of dental erosion. Aust Dent J 2003;48:97–101.
9   Addy M, Pearce N: Aetiological, predisposing and environmental factors in dentine hypersensitivity. Arch Oral Biol 1994;39(suppl):33S–38S.
10 Kaifu Y: Changes in the pattern of tooth wear from prehistoric to recent periods in Japan. Am J Phys Anthropol 1999;109:485–499.
11 Begg PR: Stone age man's dentition. Am J Orthod 1954;40:298–312, 373–383, 462–475, 517–531.
12 Kaifu Y, Kasai K, Townsend GC, Richards LC: Tooth wear and the 'design' of the human dentition: a perspective from evolutionary medicine. Am J Phys Anthropol 2003;(suppl 37): 47–61.
13 Lee R: Esthetics in relation to function; in Rufenacht CR (ed): Fundamentals in Esthetics. Chicago, Quintessence, 1990, pp 137–183.
14 McNamara JA, Seligman DA, Okeson JP: Occlusion, orthodontic treatment, and temporomandibular disorders: a review. J Orofac Pain 1995;9:73–90.
15 De Boever JA, Carlsson GE, Klineberg IJ: Need for occlusal therapy and prosthodontic treatment in the management of temporomandibular disorders. II. Tooth loss and prosthodontic treatment. J Oral Rehabil 2000;27:647–659.

16   Gesch D, Bernhardt O, Kirbschus A: Association of malocclusion and functional occlusion with temporomandibular disorders (TMD) in adults: a systematic review of population-based studies. Quintessence Int 2004;35:211–221.

17   Gesch D, Bernhardt O, Mack F, John U, Kocher T, Alte D: Association of malocclusion and functional occlusion with subjective symptoms of TMD in adults: results of the Study of Health in Pomerania (SHIP). Angle Orthod 2005;75:183–190.

18   Koh H, Robinson PJ: Occlusal adjustment for treating and preventing temporomandibular joint disorders. Cochrane Database Syst Rev 2003; Art No: CD003812, DOI: 10 1002/14651858 CD003812 2003.

19   Richards LC: Degenerative changes in the temporomandibular joint in two Australian aboriginal populations. J Dent Res 1988;67:1529–1533.

20   Richards LC: Tooth wear and temporomandibular joint change in Australian aboriginal populations. Am J Phys Anthropol 1990;82:377–384.

21   Wedel A, Borrman H, Carlsson GE: Tooth wear and temporomandibular joint morphology in a skull material from the 17th century. Swed Dent J 1998;22:85–95.

22   Owen CP, Wilding RJ, Morris AG: Changes in mandibular condyle morphology related to tooth wear in a prehistoric human population. Arch Oral Biol 1991;36:799–804.

23   Owen CP, Wilding RJ, Adams LP: Dimensions of the temporal glenoid fossa and tooth wear in prehistoric human skeletons. Arch Oral Biol 1992;37:63–67.

24   Elias AC, Sheiham A: The relationship between satisfaction with mouth and number and position of teeth. J Oral Rehabil 1998;25:649–661.

25   Rufenacht CR: Fundamentals of Esthetics. Chicago, Quintessenz, 1990.

26   Hilhorst M: Physical beauty: only skin deep? Med Health Care Philos 2002;5:11–21.

Priv.-Doz. Dr. Carolina Ganss
Department of Conservative and Preventive Dentistry
Dental Clinic, Justus Liebig University Giessen
Schlangenzahl 14, DE–35392 Giessen (Germany)

Chapter 3

Lussi A (ed): Dental Erosion.
Monogr Oral Sci. Basel, Karger, 2006, vol 20, pp 17–31

....

Interaction between Attrition, Abrasion and Erosion in Tooth Wear

M. Addy, R.P. Shellis

Applied Clinical Research Group, Bristol University Dental School, Bristol, UK

Abstract

Tooth wear is the result of three processes: abrasion (wear produced by interaction between teeth and other materials), attrition (wear through tooth–tooth contact) and erosion (dissolution of hard tissue by acidic substances). A further process (abfraction) might potentiate wear by abrasion and/or erosion. Both clinical and experimental observations show that individual wear mechanisms rarely act alone but interact with each other. The most important interaction is the potentiation of abrasion by erosive damage to the dental hard tissues. This interaction seems to be the major factor in occlusal and cervical wear. The available evidence seems insufficient to establish whether abfraction is an important contributor to tooth wear in vivo. Saliva can modulate erosive/abrasive tooth wear through formation of pellicle and by remineralisation but cannot prevent it.

In humans eating unrefined diets, the dentition eventually becomes severely worn [1]. Since the Industrial Revolution, the diet in the West has become softer and easier to masticate and this has resulted in a marked reduction in tooth wear: while postcanine teeth in modern humans wear at 15–20 µm/year [2], incisors wore at 280–360 µm/year in prehistoric humans [3]. Because tooth wear in modern Western populations is ordinarily low, pronounced wear tends to have pathological causes. The main forms of abnormal wear are cervical wear associated mainly with excessive toothbrushing, heavy occlusal wear associated with bruxism, and erosive wear at many surfaces due to ingestion of acidic substances or regurgitation of acid. This paper is concerned with the wear processes that operate in these conditions, and with their interactions to produce the clinically observable result.

The term tooth wear denotes the gradual loss of dental hard tissues through three processes: abrasion (wear produced by interaction between teeth and other materials), attrition (wear through tooth–tooth contact) and erosion (dissolution of hard tissue by acidic substances). It has been postulated that in a fourth wear-related process (abfraction) abnormal occlusal loading predisposes cervical enamel to mechanical and chemical wear [4]. All four processes are distinguished from loss of dental tissues through dental caries on the one hand and acute trauma on the other.

The terms abrasion, attrition and erosion have been adapted from everyday usage and their meanings in the dental context can diverge from those in other fields, in particular from that of tribology, the science of wear, friction and lubrication. Tribology recognises a variety of mechanisms by which wear can occur, of which the most relevant to the present paper are two- and three-body abrasion and tribochemical wear [5]. In two-body wear, two moving surfaces contact each other directly and wear is produced by breaking away of asperities. In three-body wear, two moving surfaces are separated by an intervening slurry of abrasive particles, which remove material from both surfaces. In tribochemical wear, attack by a chemical agent weakens the superficial region of the material and enhances its susceptibility to mechanical forces. Clearly, in tribological terms, attrition would be subsumed under abrasion, erosion would be described as a form of tribochemical wear and abfraction as a form of fatigue [5]. It has been suggested that the time has come to align tooth wear terminology with tribology [6] but it seems likely that the terms outlined above, most of which have had their current meaning for decades, will persist despite their limitations.

Each tooth wear process can, under some circumstances, operate alone. For example, nocturnal grinding of teeth will cause wear by attrition alone, drinking an acidic drink through a straw directed at the labial surface of the central incisors will cause wear by erosion alone, and brushing the teeth immediately on awakening will produce wear by abrasion alone. Yet, as many authors have suggested, the tooth wear observed in an individual will have resulted from a combination of all three main processes even though one may predominate [5, 7, 8]. If tooth wear were due to purely mechanical causes (abrasion and attrition), the total tissue loss at surfaces would fit a simple additive arithmetic model but wear is less simple. For example, tooth loading could create cracks which could cause particles of hard tissue to break off and act as an abrasive, thus converting a two-body attrition process into three-body abrasion [5], or the cracks would make the tissues more susceptible to abrasion, as suggested for abfraction [4]. If there is significant erosion, then the possibility of using simple arithmetic models to predict total tooth wear over time becomes remote, because erosion both removes hard tissue directly and renders tooth surfaces more susceptible to mechanical wear.

As with any oral condition which is complex even when modelled in vitro, it is always tempting to discuss the aetiology of wear without reference to the oral environment. Yet it is clear from epidemiological surveys and numerous studies in vivo, in situ and in vitro that many individual and intra-oral factors can modulate tooth wear in vivo [8–10]. Most of these are probably little understood, if at all, at this time.

In this review, we first consider the main tooth wear processes individually. We then discuss how these interact in producing clinical wear, evaluate the significance of abfraction and consider the role of saliva in modulating wear.

Tooth Wear Mechanisms

Dental Attrition

Attrition is the physiological wearing away of dental hard tissues through tooth-to-tooth contact, without the intervention of foreign substances [11]. It should in principle occur by two-body wear but mechanistically it cannot be differentiated sharply from dental abrasion, since particles of enamel detached during attrition can act as abrasive particles [12, 13].

In vitro, the rate of enamel/enamel attrition under loads of 0.2–16 kg increases with time and load, and is strongly influenced by the presence and nature of lubricant [13–15]. Above 10 kg load, water-lubricated wear is greater than between dry or saliva-lubricated surfaces but saliva-lubricated wear only exceeds wear of dry enamel at loads >14 kg [13]. Presumably, water or saline can keep detached particles of enamel in suspension and thus facilitate three-body abrasion, whereas mucins and other salivary macromolecules reduce frictional forces by coating both the wear surfaces and the particles. At loads of 6 and 10 kg, the rate of dentine/dentine attrition was found to be greater than that of enamel/enamel attrition but at 14 kg the rates were the same [16]. It was suggested that dentine wear was greater at lower loads because of its relatively low mineral content, but that at high loads the fibrous organic matrix would help to reduce fracture, whereas the more highly mineralised enamel would lack this mechanism [16].

Experimental studies of attrition to date have used loads somewhat lower than those observed during the occlusal contact phase of chewing (~27 kg [17]) and much lower than those which can occur in bruxism [18], so further experimentation using higher loads would be informative, as would studies of enamel/dentine attrition.

Clinically, occlusal wear is commonly attributed to attrition when wear on opposing teeth is equal and creates matching facets [7]. Attrition can also be involved in wear of buccal and lingual surfaces, particularly with certain malocclusions, and also interproximal surfaces. Pathological levels of attrition of occlusal surfaces, beyond the limited amount that is considered physiological, are associated with parafunctional habits, notably bruxism. However, excessive occlusal wear often seems to have a multifactorial aetiology, so is discussed later, in the context of interactions of wear mechanisms.

Dental Abrasion

Definitions sometimes assume that all dental abrasion is pathological. For example, Imfeld [11] defined abrasion as 'the pathological wearing away of dental hard tissue through abnormal mechanical processes involving foreign objects or substances repeatedly introduced in the mouth and contacting the teeth'. However, it has been suggested that many dental health problems are caused or exacerbated by almost the complete lack of abrasive wear from the diet in modern Western populations [1] and it is accepted that even normal tooth-cleaning practices produce some abrasion of dentine over a lifetime. Given that tooth-cleaning habits are highly beneficial at the same time as being the most common cause of abrasion, it would seem reasonable to remove the words pathological and abnormal from the above definition. This is not to deny that abusive use of toothbrushes and toothpaste can produce pathological levels of abrasion, as parafunction can with attrition.

In Western populations, the major abrasive agent is toothpaste, which affects dentine much more than enamel. The evidence identifying toothbrush-ing with toothpaste as the main agent in dentine abrasion is drawn from clinical data and studies in vitro [7, 19, 20, for reviews]. In toothbrushing abrasion, the toothbrush itself is merely the delivery vehicle, since brushing without paste has no effect on enamel and clinically minuscule effects on dentine [21]. Nevertheless, features of the toothbrush, notably filament arrangement, density and texture, can modulate the abrasivity of toothpaste [22, 23]. Toothbrushing wear is time-dependent and appears to be influenced by many factors, including the frequency, duration and force of brushing [19, 20]. The sites of predilection for dentine wear seem to be correlated with toothbrushing habits; the sides, teeth and sites at most risk are those known to receive most attention during brushing.

The major factor in dentine wear appears to be the relative dentine abrasiv-ity (RDA) of the toothpaste, which is its abrasivity relative to a standard paste, which has an RDA set at 100, determined using an International Standards Organisation (ISO) laboratory test. ISO stipulates that the RDA of toothpastes should not exceed 250 but most toothpastes in developed countries have RDA ≤ 100. Difficulties arise in extrapolating RDA to clinical outcome. Philpotts et al. [24] observed a close linear relationship between RDA and dentine wear in vitro but in situ, although increasing RDA tends to be associated with greater wear, the relationship is much less clear cut [25–27]. In addition, there is often considerable variability in measurements of wear in situ [25, 27].

Only dentifrices with high relative enamel abrasivities (REA) cause appreciable rates of enamel wear, usually because they use non-hydrated alumina, which is harder than enamel. Dentifrices with relative enamel abrasivities <10 produce very little wear of enamel in vitro or in situ [24, 26–29].

It has been concluded that normal toothbrushing habits with toothpastes that conform with the ISO standard will, in a lifetime's use, cause virtually no wear of enamel and clinically insignificant abrasion of dentine (a figure of 1 mm in around 100 years is often cited [19, 20]).

Dental Erosion

Dental erosion is the loss of tooth structure by acid dissolution without the involvement of bacteria. The acids may be intrinsic (regurgitated gastric acid) or extrinsic (acidic industrial vapours or dietary components such as soft drinks, pickles, acidic fruits). Epidemiological data, and studies in vitro and in situ, suggest that, of the three individual wear processes, erosion is the most common threat for tooth surface loss [9, 10]. Most erosion research has been concerned with enamel but there is a growing interest in dentine, perhaps encouraged by evidence that dentine hypersensitivity appears to be a tooth wear phenomenon [30].

Enamel exposed to acid loses mineral from a layer extending a few micrometres below the surface: a process known as softening [31]. With time, as softening progresses further into the enamel, dissolution in the most superficial enamel will reach the point where this layer of enamel is lost completely [32, 33]. In vivo, erosion could therefore involve two types of wear of enamel: the direct removal of hard tissue by complete dissolution and the creation of a thin softened layer, which is vulnerable to subsequent mechanical wear (see chapter 6 by Featherstone et al., this vol, pp 66–76). The pH fall at tooth surfaces following a single ingestion of an acidic drink seems to be fairly short-lived [34] and likely to produce softening, but repeated intake of erosive drinks might favour more advanced demineralisation consistent with total tissue loss.

The mineral content of enamel from deciduous teeth is lower than in permanent teeth but the two seem to be equally susceptible to erosion in vitro [35–37]. In situ, the enamel of deciduous teeth becomes more susceptible than that of permanent teeth at a high frequency of acid exposure ($4\times$/day) [38].

In dentine exposed to acid there is first dissolution at the junction of the peritubular and intertubular dentine, then loss of the peritubular dentine and widening of the tubule lumina [39] and finally formation of a superficial layer of demineralised collagenous matrix [40]. While it persists, this layer might mechanically protect the underlying residual dentine and might also affect chemical reactions between the latter and the oral fluids, but it is itself vulnerable to mechanical and proteolytic damage and will ultimately be lost. Hunter et al. [36] found no difference in susceptibility to erosion of dentine from deciduous and permanent teeth in vitro but, in situ, dentine from deciduous teeth was less susceptible at a high frequency of acid exposure (4×/day) [38].

Erosion in vitro and in situ is influenced by biological variation within dental tissues. Clinically there is clear inter-subject variation. It is likely that the flow rate, electrolyte composition, buffer capacity and protein composition of saliva contribute strongly to this variability, by influencing the rate at which saliva recovers from undersaturation following an acid challenge [41] and by determining the remineralisation potential [42]. The suggestion that the thickness and protective properties of the salivary pellicle influence site variations in erosion [43] does not seem to be supported experimentally [44].

Interactions between Tooth Wear Processes

It is well-recognised that interactions between different mechanisms contribute strongly to clinically-observed patterns of wear. However, it is difficult in many cases either to determine the major cause of wear or to evaluate how different wear mechanisms have interacted. There is a consensus that interactions between mechanical and erosive wear are the most important in vivo and these have been the subject of a number of laboratory investigations. We describe these studies as a preliminary to considering clinical studies. It is appropriate also to discuss here the theory of abfraction, as it might potentiate other wear mechanisms.

Interaction of Dental Attrition with Erosion

At loads up to 16 kg, enamel/enamel attrition in vitro is much higher in the presence of HCl (pH 1.2) than in water [14]. However, this extreme erosive challenge is likely to occur in vivo only in individuals who vomit frequently, e.g. bulimics [45]. Attrition is much lower in the presence of dilute acetic acid (pH 3.0) or citric acid (pH 3.2), which are much closer to more usual erosive stimuli, than in the presence of water or saline [13–15]. Enamel surfaces which had been rubbed together in citric acid solution at pH 3.2 were smooth, with only slight grooving, and it was suggested that acid softening would both reduce friction between the surfaces and also dissolve potentially abrasive enamel particles fractured off the surfaces [13]. Studies of enamel surfaces worn by attrition under higher loads, more representative of chewing or bruxism, and in the presence and absence of acid, would be of interest. There have been no controlled in vitro studies of dentine attrition under acidic conditions.

Interaction of Dental Abrasion with Erosion

Exposure of enamel to acid renders it more vulnerable to abrasion. Rats drinking an acidic drink instead of water showed occlusal and lingual wear of the molars, whether they were consuming soft or hard food [46]. In vitro, softened enamel is more susceptible to abrasion, not only by toothbrush and paste [47–49], but even by such mild challenges as toothbrushing without paste [50] or friction from the tongue [51]. Thus, whereas enamel is scarcely abraded by normal toothbrushing, it becomes vulnerable to toothbrush abrasion after erosive challenge (see chapter 12 by Lussi et al., this vol, pp 190–199).

There is a gradient of mineral loss in softened enamel [52, 53] and the outer extremities of the crystals are thinned and would be extremely vulnerable to mechanical forces [53]. A physical challenge probably removes only the outer, more demineralised part of the softened enamel to leave the inner, less demineralised part [53]. It can be conjectured that abraded softened enamel surfaces would be more susceptible to fresh acid challenges, but this has yet to be tested experimentally. It was found that brushing simultaneously with exposure to citric acid enhanced wear by about 50% compared with brushing after acid exposure [50]. The increase is probably due to a primarily increased rate of mineral dissolution because of increased fluid movement [50, 54], which will result in more rapid creation and breakage of thinned crystal extremities.

Several studies have shown that acid-softened dentine is also vulnerable to toothbrush abrasion, both in vitro [47, 55] and in situ [56, 57].

Abfraction

The principal idea in the theory of abfraction, which was proposed to account for the creation of wedge-shaped non-carious cervical lesions [58], is that off-axis loading of tooth cusps would cause tensile stress concentrations in the cervical region, leading to micro-crack formation, particularly in the enamel, which resists tensile stress less well than dentine. The weakened cervical region would then be susceptible to abrasion and erosion [4, 6].

The evidence for abfraction as an important factor in tooth wear seems to be inconclusive [59]. In particular, there seems to be no firm clinical evidence for the phenomenon. There are also problems with non-clinical studies. While a number of analyses of stress distributions in loaded teeth support the concept of cervical stress concentrations, many have used unrealistic models of tooth structure or have yielded results that conflict with the predictions of the abfraction hypothesis [60]. Wedge-shaped cervical lesions can be created in vitro by brushing teeth that are either unloaded or under continuous axial load [61]. Moreover, while axial loading reduced cervical toothbrushing wear, off-axis loading had no significant effect [61]. It is always possible that experiments on extracted teeth are influenced by preexisting cracks in the cervical enamel but these results cast doubt on the validity of the abfraction hypothesis. Periodic off-axis stressing of whole tooth crowns increased the rate of erosion of cervical enamel in 1% lactic acid, pH 4.5 [62], but in this study only tissue loss on the crown surface subject to tensile stress was examined and examination of both surfaces is essential to test the abfraction hypothesis. Staninec et al. [63] found that tissue loss from beams of dentine subjected to bending stress was greater at pH 6 than at pH 7, but more wear occurred on the compression surface of the beam than on the tension surface and this is contradictory to the abfraction hypothesis.

In an interesting finite-element study [64], it was predicted that a discontinuity at the enamel–dentine junction in the cervical region could create stress concentrations that would exceed the breaking strength of enamel. In vivo such a discontinuity could be created by cervical erosion or root-surface caries and need not involve enamel demineralisation, because of the solubility difference between enamel and dentine.

Clinical Observations

At present, it is difficult to determine the importance in vivo of the processes discussed in the foregoing, for several reasons. Much of the evidence for interaction between wear processes in clinical tooth wear comes mainly from case reports, which can only suggest associations between different wear mechanisms and are inconclusive as to their interactions. Clinical and epidemiological studies of tooth wear tend to concentrate on one wear process. Thus, while there are many excellent studies of erosion, they have concentrated largely on the acids responsible for erosion, although, some information about the possible role of such factors as toothbrushing habits has been gathered. Most epidemiological studies on tooth wear have been cross-sectional but, since wear accumulates over a long period, it is difficult or impossible to tease out the impact of individual wear processes in the overall wear. More case-control studies or, better still, longitudinal studies could provide more conclusive evidence. Studies of this type, concentrating on individuals exposed to a dominant wear process, should yield data that allow the effect of that process on clinical wear, while taking into account oral hygiene and dietary, medical and other factors. There may be some scope for improving methods for examining clinical wear. For instance, examination of replicas by SEM [65] can provide more details of wear patterns for research purposes. Indirect indicators of tooth wear, such as the presence and severity of dentine hypersensitivity, could be useful. Notwithstanding these comments, some knowledge of interacting wear processes has been gained.

Occlusal Wear

Several studies have found that occlusal wear may be related to a variety of factors, including occlusal variations, dusty environments, salivary variables and intake of acidic foods and drinks [66–68]. These observations suggest that erosion, abrasion or both probably contribute to occlusal wear. From detailed observation of tooth surfaces it was concluded that erosion was a major factor in heavy occlusal wear in one Australian sample, except in anterior teeth of positively-identified bruxers [65]. The limited in vitro data suggest that erosive softening of dental tissues is likely to increase abrasive wear but not attritional wear. This is consistent with the finding [46] that the total amount of wear on molars of rats drinking an erosive liquid did not depend on the hardness of the food. Persons subsisting on a raw-food diet, which was both fibrous and with a high acid content, developed marked occlusal wear, with cupping of the exposed dentine [69]. The similarity of the pattern of wear to that in a mediaeval population with an abrasive diet suggested that an erosive diet softens the occlusal surfaces and makes them vulnerable to wear even by weakly abrasive materials, such as raw vegetables, which would not affect sound dentine [70].

An index for assessing clinical wear and for predicting the future rate of wear would be useful. Information on tooth wear in relation to age exists for various populations, mostly historical [71]. Richards et al. [72] used such data to develop a mathematical model of the normal progression of wear with age. While this approach has great potential, its successful application in a particular population requires that the wear data on which it is based are derived from the same population or one very like it.

Cervical Wear

The most common sites for abnormal tooth wear are the buccal cervical regions and there has been considerable interest in the aetiology of this wear process, thoroughly reviewed by Levitch et al. [73]. Obviously, a direct role for attrition in creation of these lesions can be ruled out. Recognition of the synergy between erosion and mechanical wear has led most researchers to consider these to be erosion/abrasion lesions rather than the often-described cervical abrasion lesions. Erosion must be a factor in any lesion involving enamel since, as discussed above, most modern dentifrices produce very little wear of enamel.

The abfraction hypothesis has drawn attention to the possibility that unusual occlusal loads, resulting from tooth misalignment or heavy muscular force, may be associated with non-carious cervical lesions, but the evidence for this is not conclusive. Studies which considered cervical lesion characteristics in relation to occlusal wear or malocclusion [74, 75] suggest that the proportion of lesions possibly due to abfraction was 15–38%. Khan et al. [76] found saucer-shaped lesions to be associated strongly with occlusal erosion, while wedge-shaped lesions were associated equally with occlusal erosion and attrition. Cervical lesions of all kinds were much more prevalent in persons eating an erosive raw-food diet than in controls, but were absent in a sample of mediaeval dentitions with heavy occlusal wear [69, 70]. However, the latter could be due to reduced eccentric loading or other causes [70]. In a case-control study [77], only variables considered to be related to abrasion were significant risk factors for cervical lesions in a subject-level model, while variables related to tooth flexure and erosion were also significant risk factors in a tooth-level model. In summary, the evidence suggests that non-carious cervical lesions have a multifactorial aetiology, with combined erosion and abrasion probably playing the dominant role.

Saliva and Tooth Wear

The importance of saliva as a lubricant has been alluded to above [14]. Saliva is also the source of the acquired pellicle, which reduces the amount of mineral loss in short-term erosion. However, during acid exposure, the pellicle is removed except for the dense basal layer and its protective effect is lost [44, 78]. Thus, to determine whether pellicle protects against repeated erosive and abrasive challenges it is important to determine how quickly the protective effect is re-established. In vitro tests indicate that a significant protective effect is achieved after exposure to saliva for 2 min for dentine and 1 h for enamel [79].

The pellicle seems to show some resistance to brushing, since the basal pellicle layer survives 10 s brushing with saliva alone [80]. Brushing with hydrated alumina or saliva/silica slurry was reported to leave a thin pellicle layer on enamel [80, 81] and Hannig [80] suggested that this layer could modify wear. However, brushing with these abrasives would cause no significant wear of sound enamel and this hypothesis needs to be tested using softened enamel. Moreover, the finding that brushing removes the outer pellicle [80] substantiates the suggestion [82] that brushing immediately before eating or drinking might reduce the protective effect of the pellicle against erosion (see chapter 12 by Lussi et al., this vol, pp 190–199).

Softened enamel exposed to a remineralising solution or to saliva for an adequate time can regain mineral and thus re-acquire mechanical strength [31, 52, 83–85]. In vivo saliva could thus reduce the vulnerability of softened dental hard tissues to mechanical wear. In vitro, resistance to toothbrush abrasion [84] or to ultrasonication [85] was restored after exposure to artificial saliva for 4 and 6 h, respectively. In vivo results over times that would be useful in terms of reducing abrasion of softened enamel have been less encouraging. In one in situ experiment, only partial resistance to brushing abrasion was acquired after 60 min exposure to saliva [49], while in another the decrease in abrasion after the same time was not significant [82]. The discrepancy between the in vitro and in situ results might be due to the presence in saliva of proteins (e.g. statherins) known to inhibit hydroxyapatite crystal growth, and their absence from the artificial salivas used in in vitro experiments.

As regards dentine, exposure to saliva seems to be ineffective in restoring abrasion resistance within a useful time. In vitro exposure to artificial saliva for up to 2 h [55] or for 24 h [86] produced no improvement in resistance to subsequent mechanical challenge. One in situ study showed no effect on abrasion resistance after exposure to saliva for 1 h [56]. In another there was a numerical decrease in abrasion resistance after 30 and 60 min remineralisation [57] but in neither case was the tissue loss significantly different from that in specimens brushed immediately after erosion. While artificial caries lesions of dentine can be remineralised in vitro [87], it is not complete even after 20 weeks, and remineralisation of such lesions seems to take place by re-growth of residual mineral crystals. In erosive dentine lesions, the superficial layer seems to be completely demineralised and Clarkson et al. [88] showed that dentine demineralised by organic acids does not remineralise because it retains phosphoproteins which may act as inhibitors.

References

1   Kaifu Y, Kasai, K, Townsend GC, Richards LC: Tooth wear and the 'design' of the human dentition: a perspective from evolutionary medicine. Yearb Phys Anthropol 2003;46:47–61.
2   Lambrechts P, Braem M, Vuylsteke-Wauters M, Vanherle G: Quantitative in vivo wear of human enamel. J Dent Res 1989;68:1752–1754.
3   Bermúdez de Castro JM, Martinón-Torres M, Sarmiento S, Lozano M, Arsuaga JL, Carbonell E: Rates of anterior tooth wear in Middle Pleistocene hominins from Sima de los Huesos (Sierra de Atapuerca, Spain). Proc Natl Acad Sci USA 2003;100:11992–11996.
4   Grippo JO: Abfractions: a new classification of hard tissue lesions of teeth. J Esthet Dent 1991;3:14–19.
5   Mair LH: Wear in the mouth: the tribological dimension; in Addy M, Embery G, Edgar WM, Orchardson R (eds): Tooth Wear and Sensitivity. London, Martin Dunitz, 2000, pp 181–188.
6   Grippo JO, Simring M, Schreiner S: Attrition, abrasion, corrosion and abfraction revisited. J Am Dent Assoc 2004;135:1109–1117.

7   Bartlett D, Smith BGN: Definition, classification, and clinical assessment of attrition, erosion and abrasion of enamel and dentine; in Addy M, Embery G, Edgar WM, Orchardson R (eds): Tooth Wear and Sensitivity. London, Martin Dunitz, 2000, pp 87–92.

8   Meurman JH, Sorvari R: Interplay of erosion attrition and abrasion in toothwear and possible approaches to prevention; in Addy M, Embery G, Edgar WM, Orchardson R (eds): Tooth Wear and Sensitivity. London, Martin Dunitz, 2000, pp 171–180.

9   Nunn JH: Prevalence and distribution of tooth wear; in Addy M, Embery G, Edgar WM, Orchardson R (eds): Tooth Wear and Sensitivity. London, Martin Dunitz, 2000, pp 93–104.

10 Zero DT, Lussi A: Etiology of enamel erosion: intrinsic and extrinsic factors; in Addy M, Embery G, Edgar WM, Orchardson R (eds): Tooth Wear and Sensitivity. London, Martin Dunitz, 2000, pp 121–140.

11 Imfeld T: Dental erosion. Definition, classification and links. Eur J Oral Sci 1996;104:151–155.

12 Xhonga FA: Bruxism and its effect on the teeth. J Oral Rehabil 1977;4:65–76.

13 Eisenburger M, Addy M: Erosion and attrition of human enamel in vitro. I. Interaction effects. J Dent 2002;30:341–347.

14 Kaidonis JA, Richards LC, Townsend GC, Tansley GD: Wear of human enamel: a quantitative assessment. J Dent Res 1998;77:1983–1990.

15 Eisenburger M, Addy M: Erosion and attrition of human enamel in vitro. II. Influence of time and loading. J Dent 2002;30:349–352.

16 Burak N, Kaidonis JA, Richards LC, Townsend GC: Experimental studies of human dentine wear. Arch Oral Biol 1999;44:885–885.

17 Gibbs CH, Mahan PE, Lundeen HC, Brehnan K, Walsh EK, Holbrook WB: Occlusal forces during chewing and swallowing as measured by sound transmission. J Prosthet Dent 1981;46:443–449.

18 Waltimo A, Nyström M, Könönen M: Bite force and dentofacial morphology in men with severe dental attrition. Scand J Dent Res 1994;102:92–96.

19 Addy M, Hunter ML: Can toothbrushing damage your health? Effects on oral and dental tissues. Int Dent J 2003;53:177–186.

20 Hunter ML, Addy M, Pickles MJ, Joiner A: The role of toothpastes and toothbrushes in the aetiology of toothwear. Int Dent J 2002;52:399–405.

21 Absi EG, Addy M, Adams D: Dentine hypersensitivity. The effects of toothbrushing and dietary compounds on dentine in vitro: a SEM study. J Oral Rehabil 1992;19:101–110.

22 Phaneuf EA, Harrington JH, Dale PP, Shklar G: Automatic toothbrush: a new reciprocating action. J Am Dent Assoc 1962;65:12–25.

23 Dyer D, Addy M, Newcombe RG: Studies in vitro of abrasion by different manual toothbrush heads and a standard toothpaste. J Clin Periodontol 2000;27:99–103.

24 Philpotts CJ, Weader E, Joiner A: The measurement in vitro of enamel and dentine wear by toothpastes of different abrasivity. Int Dent J 2005;55:183–187.

25 Addy M, Hughes J, Pickles M, Joiner A, Huntington E: Development of a method in situ to study toothpaste abrasion of dentine: comparison of 2 products. J Clin Periodontol 2002;29: 896–900.

26 Hooper SM, West NX, Pickles MJ, Joiner A, Newcombe RG, Addy M: Investigation of erosion and abrasion of enamel and dentine: a model in situ using toothpastes of different abrasivity. J Clin Periodontol 2003;30:802–808.

27 Pickles MJ, Joiner A, Weader E, Cooper YL, Cox TF: Abrasion of human enamel and dentine caused by toothpastes of differing abrasivity determined using an in situ wear model. Int Dent J 2005;55:188–193.

28 Joiner A, Pickles MJ, Tanner C, Weader E, Doyle P: An in situ model to study the toothpaste abrasion of enamel. J Clin Periodontol 2004;31:434–438.

29 Lussi A, Jaeggi T, Gerber C, Megert B: Effect of amine/sodium fluoride rinsing on toothbrush abrasion of softened enamel in situ. Caries Res 2004;38:567–571.

30 Dababneh RH, Khouri AT, Addy M: Dentine hypersensitivity – an enigma? A review of terminology, epidemiology, mechanisms, aetiology and management. Br Dent J 1999;187:606–611.

31 Koulourides T: Experimental changes of mineral density; in Harris RS (ed): Art and Science of Dental Caries Research. New York, Academic Press, 1968, pp 355–378.

32 Schweizer-Hirt CM, Schait A, Schmidt R, Imfeld T, Lutz F, Mühlemann HR: Erosion und Abrasion des Schmelzes: eine experimentelle Studie. Schweiz Monatsschr Zahnheilkd 1978;88:497–529.

33 Eisenburger M, Hughes J, West NX, Jandt K, Addy M: Ultrasonication as a method to study enamel demineralization during acid erosion. Caries Res 2000;34:289–294.

34 Millward A, Shaw L, Harrington E, Smith AJ: Continuous monitoring of salivary flow rate and pH at the surface of the dentition following consumption of acidic beverages. Caries Res 1997;31: 44–49.

35 Lussi A, Kohler N, Zero D, Schaffner M, Megert B: A comparison of the erosive potential of different beverages in primary and permanent teeth using an in vitro model. Eur J Oral Sci 2000;108: 110–114.

36 Hunter ML, West NX, Hughes JA, Newcombe RG, Addy M: Relative susceptibility of deciduous and permanent dental hard tissues to erosion by a low pH fruit drink in vitro. J Dent 2000;28: 265–270.

37 Johansson A-K, Sorvari R, Birkhed D, Meurman JH: Dental erosion in deciduous teeth – an in vivo and in vitro study. J Dent 2001;29:333–340.

38 Hunter ML, West NX, Hughes JA, Newcombe RG, Addy M: Erosion of deciduous and permanent dental hard tissue in the oral environment. J Dent 2000;28:257–263.

39 Meurman JH, Drysdale T, Frank RM: Experimental erosion of dentine. Scand J Dent Res 1991;99:457–462.

40 Kinney JH, Balooch M, Haupt DL, Marshall SJ, Marshall GW: Mineral distribution and dimensional changes in human dentine during demineralization. J Dent Res 1995;74:1179–1184.

41 Bashir E, Lagerlöf F: Effect of citric acid clearance on the saturation with respect to hydroxyapatite in saliva. Caries Res 1996;30:213–217.

42 Amaechi BT, Higham SM: Eroded enamel lesion remineralization by saliva as a possible factor in the site-specificity of human dental erosion. Arch Oral Biol 2001;46:697–703.

43 Amaechi BT, Higham SM: Thickness of acquired salivary pellicle as a determinant of the sites of dental erosion. J Dent Res 1999;78:1821–1828.

44 Hannig M, Balz M: Protective properties of salivary pellicles from two different intraoral sites on enamel erosion. Caries Res 2001;35:142–148.

45 Järvinen VK, Rytömaa II, Heinonen OP: Risk factors in dental erosion. J Dent Res 1991;70:942–947.

46 Sorvari R, Kiviranta I: A semiquantitative method of recording experimental tooth erosion and estimating occlusal wear in the rat. Arch Oral Biol 1988;33:217–220.

47 Davis WB, Winter PJ: The effect of abrasion on enamel and dentine after exposure to dietary acid. Br Dent J 1980;148:253–256.

48 Attin T, Koidl, Buchalla W, Schaller HG, Kielbassa AM, Hellwig E: Correlation of microhardness and wear in differently eroded bovine dental enamel. Arch Oral Biol 1996;42:243–250.

49 Jaeggi T, Lussi A: Toothbrush abrasion of erosively altered enamel after intraoral exposure to saliva: an in situ study. Caries Res 1999;33:455–461.

50 Eisenburger M, Shellis RP, Addy M: Comparative study of wear of enamel induced by alternating and simultaneous combinations of abrasion and erosion in vitro. Caries Res 2003;37:450–456.

51 Gregg T, Mace S, West NX, Addy M: A study in vitro of the abrasive effect of the tongue on enamel and dentine softened by acid erosion. Caries Res 2004;38:557–560.

52 Amaechi BT, Higham SM: In vitro remineralization of eroded enamel lesions by saliva. J Dent 2001;29:371–376.

53 Eisenburger M, Shellis RP, Addy M: Scanning electron microscopy of softened enamel. Caries Res 2004;38:67–74.

54 Shellis RP, Finke M, Eisenburger M, Parker DM, Addy M: Relationship between enamel erosion and flow rate. Eur J Oral Sci 2005;113:232–238.

55 Attin T, Buchalla W, Putz B: In vitro evaluation of different remineralization periods in improving the abrasion resistance of previously abraded bovine dentine against tooth-brushing abrasion. Arch Oral Biol 2001;46:871–874.

56 Hara AT, Turssi CP, Teixeira EC, Serra MC, Cury JA: Abrasive wear on eroded root dentine after different periods of exposure to saliva in situ. Eur J Oral Sci 2003;111:423–427.

57 Attin T, Siegel S, Buchalla W, Lennon ÁM, Hannig C, Becker K: Brushing abrasion of softened and remineralised dentin: an in situ study. Caries Res 2004;38:62–66.

58   Lee WC, Eakles WS: Possible role of tensile stress in the etiology of cervical erosive lesions of the teeth. J Prosthet Dent 1984;52:374–380.

59   Litonjua LA, Andreana S, Bush PJ, Tobias TS, Cohen RE: Noncarious cervical lesions and abfractions. A re-evaluation. J Am Dent Assoc 2003;134:845–850.

60   Litonjua LA, Andreana S, Patra AK, Cohen RE: An assessment of stress analyses in the theory of abfraction. Biomed Mater Eng 2004;14:311–321.

61   Litonjua LA, Bush PJ, Andreana S, Tobias TS, Cohen RE: Effects of occlusal load on cervical lesions. J Oral Rehabil 2004;31:225–232.

62   Palamara D, Palamara JEA, Tyas MJ, Pintado M, Messer HH: Effect of stress on acid dissolution of enamel. Dent Mater 2001;17:109–115.

63   Staninec M, Nalla RK, Hilton JF, Ritchie RO, Watanabe LG, Nonomura G, Marshall GW, Marshall SJ: Dentin erosion simulation by cantilever beam fatigue and pH change. J Dent Res 2005;84:371–375.

64   Rees JS, Hammadeh M: Undermining of enamel as a mechanism of abfraction lesion formation: a finite element study. Eur J Oral Sci 2004;112:347–352.

65   Khan F, Young WG, Daley TJ: Dental erosion and bruxism. A tooth wear analysis. Aust Dent J 1998;43:117–127.

66   Nyström M, Könen M, Alaluusua S, Evälahti M, Vartiovaara J: Development of horizontal tooth wear in maxillary anterior teeth from five to 18 years of age. J Dent Res 1990;69:1765–1770.

67   Johansson A, Fareed K, Omar R: Analysis of possible factors influencing the occurrence of occlusal tooth wear in a young Saudi population. Acta Odontol Scand 1991;49:139–145.

68   Johansson A, Kiliaridis S, Haraldson T, Omar R, Carlsson GE: Covariation of some factors associated with occlusal tooth wear in a selected high-wear sample. Scand J Dent Res 1993;101: 398–406.

69   Ganss C, Schlechtriemen M, Klimek J: Dental erosions in subjects living on a raw food diet. Caries Res 1999;33:74–80.

70   Ganss, C, Klimek J, Borkovski N: Characteristics of tooth wear in relation to different nutritional patterns including contemporary and medieval subjects. Eur J Oral Sci 2002;110:54–60.

71   Miles AEW: The Miles method of assessing age from tooth wear revisited. J Archaeol Sci 2001;28:973–982.

72   Richards LC, Kaidonis JA, Townsend GC: A model for the prediction of tooth wear in individuals. Aust Dent J 2003;48:259–262.

73   Levitch LC, Bader JD, Shugars DA, Heymann HO: Non-carious cervical lesions. J Dent 1994;22: 195–207.

74   Piotrowski BT, Gillette WB, Hancock EB: Examining the prevalence and characteristics of abfraction-like cervical lesions in a population of US veterans. J Am Dent Assoc 2001;132:1694–1701.

75   Oginni AO, Olusile AO, Udoye CI: Non-carious cervical lesions in a Nigerian population: abrasion or abfraction? Int Dent J 2003;53:275–279.

76   Khan F, Young WG, Shahabi S, Daley TJ: Dental cervical lesions associated with occlusal erosion and attrition. Aust Dent J 1999;44:176–186.

77   Bader JD, McClure F, Scurria MS, Shugars DA, Heymann HO: Case-control study of non-carious cervical lesions. Community Dent Oral Epidemiol 1996;24:286–291.

78   Hannig M, Balz M: Influence of in vivo formed salivary pellicle on enamel erosion. Caries Res 1999;33:372–379.

79   Wetton S, Hughes JA, West NX, Addy M: Exposure time of enamel and dentine to saliva for protection against erosion: a study in vitro. Caries Res, in press.

80   Hannig M: The protective nature of the salivary pellicle. Int Dent J 2002;52:417–423.

81   Saxton CA: The effects of dentifrices on the appearance of the tooth surface observed with the scanning electron microscope. J Periodontal Res 1976;11:74–85.

82   Attin T, Knöfel S, Buchalla W, Tütüncü R: In situ evaluation of different remineralization periods to decrease brushing abrasion of demineralized enamel. Caries Res 2001;35:216–222.

83   Collys K, Cleymaet R, Coomans D, Michotte Y, Slop D: Rehardening of surface softened and surface etched enamel in vitro and by intraoral exposure. Caries Res 1993;27:15–20.

84   Attin T, Buchalla W, Gollner, Hellwig E: Use of variable remineralization periods to improve the abrasion resistance of previously eroded enamel. Caries Res 2000;34:48–52.

85   Eisenburger M, Addy M, Hughes JA, Shellis RP: Effect of time on the remineralization of enamel after citric acid erosion. Caries Res 2001;35:211–215.

86   Vanuspong W, Eisenburger M, Addy M: Cervical tooth wear and sensitivity: erosion, softening and rehardening of dentine: effects of pH, time and ultrasonication. J Clin Periodontol 2002;29: 351–357.

87   Mukai Y, ten Cate JM: Remineralization of advanced root dentin lesions in vitro. Caries Res 2002;36:275–280.

88   Clarkson BH, Feagin FF, McCurdy SP, Sheetz JH, Speirs RL: Effects of phosphoprotein moieties on the remineralization of human root caries. Caries Res 1991;25:166–173.

Prof. M. Addy
Restorative Dentistry (Perio)
University of Bristol Hospital and School, Lower Maudlin Street
Bristol BS1 2LY (UK)

Lussi A (ed): Dental Erosion.
Monogr Oral Sci. Basel, Karger, 2006, vol 20, pp 32–43

·····················

Diagnosis of Erosive Tooth Wear

C. Ganss[a], *A. Lussi*[b]

[a]Department of Conservative and Preventive Dentistry, Dental Clinic
Justus Liebig University Giessen, Germany; [b]Department of Preventive,
Restorative and Pediatric Dentistry, School of Dental Medicine,
University of Bern, Bern, Switzerland

Abstract

The clinical diagnosis 'erosion' is made from characteristic deviations from the original
anatomical tooth morphology, thus, distinguishing acid induced tissue loss from other forms
of wear. Primary pathognomonic features are shallow concavities on smooth surfaces occurring coronal from the enamel–cementum junction. Problems from diagnosing occlusal surfaces and exposed dentine are discussed. Indices for recording erosive wear include
morphological as well as quantitative criteria. Currently, various indices are used making the
comparison of prevalence studies difficult. The most important and frequently used indices
are described. In addition to recording erosive lesions, the assessment of progression is
important as the indication of treatment measures depends on erosion activity. A number of
evaluated and sensitive methods for in vitro and in situ approaches are available, but the fun-
damental problem for their clinical use is the lack of re-identifiable reference areas. Tools for
clinical monitoring are described.

Current Approach to Erosive Tooth Wear

'Diagnosis is the intellectual course that integrates information obtained
by clinical examination of the teeth, use of diagnostic aids, conversation with
the patient and biological knowledge. A proper diagnosis cannot be performed
without inspecting the teeth and their immediate surroundings' [1]. This definition formulated for caries is also true for erosive tooth wear. It means that a grid
pattern of criteria is pelted over the patient and thereafter the signs and symptoms are first ordered and then classified in the second step. In the same
process, the native tooth anatomy and morphology memorized engram-like is
compared with the actual appearance.

The different chemical and physical insults on teeth cause loss of dental hard tissue with some characteristic patterns. The classification of wear is made from clinically observed morphological features. However, some indices do assume information as to the etiology such as attrition, abrasion and erosion. This approach is open to debate for two reasons: (1) an association between defect morphology and the respective etiological factors has not been validly established, and (2) the presumed etiology predetermines scientific strategies and could introduce bias. It has therefore been argued that assessing wear as the super ordinate phenomenon disregarding the shape of lesions would overcome these disadvantages [2]. It is, however, important to note that the tissue loss ceases from progression when the cause is eliminated. Therefore, on a patient level it is a prerequisite to detect the condition early, to distinguish it from other defects and to search for the main cause in order to start the adequate preventive measures. From a clinical as well as from a scientific point of view, it would be necessary to have differentiating diagnostic criteria available.

Morphology and Differential Diagnosis of Erosive Tooth Wear

The early signs of erosive tooth wear appear as a smooth silky-shining glazed surface. In the more advanced stages changes in the original morphology occur (figs. 1–9).

On smooth surfaces, the convex areas flatten or concavities become present, the width of which clearly exceeds its depth. Undulating borders of the lesion are possible. Initial lesions are located coronal from the enamel–cementum junction with an intact border of enamel along the gingival margin. The reason for the preserved enamel band could be due to some plaque remnants, which act as a diffusion barrier for acids or due to an acid-neutralizing effect of the sulcular fluid, which has a pH between 7.5 and 8.0 [3]. Further acid attacks can lead to pseudo-chamfers at the margin of the eroded surface (figs. 1–3, 8, 9).

Erosion can be distinguished from wedge-shaped defects, which are located at or apical to the enamel–cementum junction. The coronal part of wedge-shaped defects ideally has a sharp margin and cuts at right angles into the enamel surface, whereas the apical part bottoms out to the root surface. The depth of the defect clearly exceeds its width.

The initial features of erosion on occlusal and incisal surfaces are the same as described above. Further progression of occlusal erosion leads to a rounding of the cusps, grooves on the cusps and incisal edges, and restorations rising above the level of the adjacent tooth surfaces. In severe cases the whole occlusal

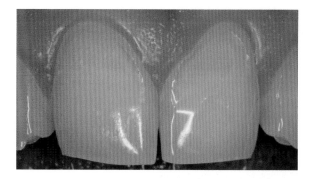

Fig. 1. Facial erosive tooth wear. Note the intact enamel along the gingival margin and the silky-glazed appearance of the tooth. Age of patient: 28 years. Known etiological factors: acidic drinks, gastroesophageal reflux.

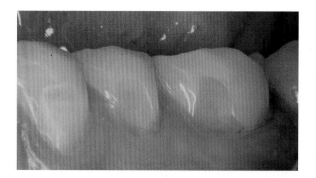

Fig. 2. Facial erosive tooth wear. No intact enamel along the gingival margin, but a silky-glazed appearance of the surface. Age of patient: 35 years. Known etiological factors: acidic fruits (lemon, orange) and fresh squeezed lemon and orange juice.

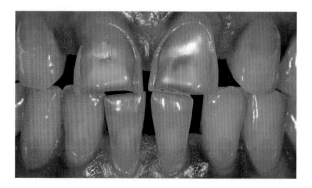

Fig. 3. Severe facial erosive tooth wear. Age of patient: 25 years. Known etiological factors: lemon slices under the lip, fruit juices.

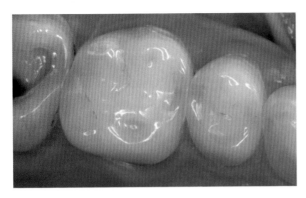

Fig. 4. Occlusal erosive tooth wear. Note rounding of the cusps and grooves. Age of patient: 29 years. Known etiological factors: soft drinks, sipping of 0.5-l acidic sports drinks per day.

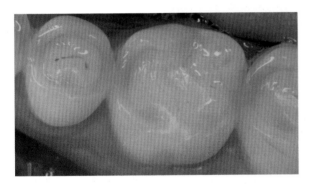

Fig. 5. Occlusal erosive tooth wear. Age of patient: 29 years (same patient as in fig. 4). The signs of erosive tooth wear are more pronounced. Known etiological factors: soft drinks, sipping of 0.5-l acidic sports drinks per day.

morphology disappears (figs. 4–7). Erosive lesions have to be distinguished from attrition. They are often flat and have glossy areas with distinct margins and corresponding features at the antagonistic teeth. Much more difficult is the distinction between occlusal erosion and abrasion/demastication, which sometimes are of similar shape.

Whenever possible, the clinical examination should be accomplished by a thorough history taking with respect to general health, diet and habits and by the assessment of saliva flow rates (see chapter 12 by Lussi et al., this vol, pp 190–199).

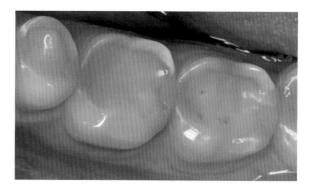

Fig. 6. Severe occlusal erosive tooth wear. No occlusal morphology present. Age of patient: 29 years. Known etiological factor: gastroesophageal reflux.

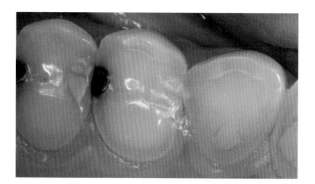

Fig. 7. Severe oral and occlusal erosive tooth wear. Note the worn oral cusps and the amalgam filling rising above the level of the adjacent tooth surface. Age of patient: 29 years (same patient as in fig. 6). Known etiological factor: gastroesophageal reflux.

Indices

Erosive tooth wear from a clinical view is a surface phenomenon, occurring on areas accessible to visual diagnosis. The diagnostic procedure is therefore a visual rather than instrumental approach.

A number of indices for the clinical diagnosis of erosive tooth wear have been proposed [4–10], which more or less are modifications or combinations of the indices published by Eccles [11] and Smith and Knight [12] (table 1). All erosion indices include diagnostic criteria to differentiate erosions from other

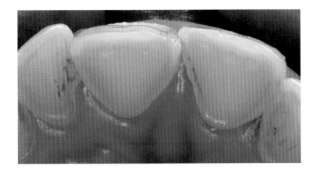

Fig. 8. Severe oral erosive tooth wear. Note the intact enamel along the gingival margin. Age of patient: 28 years. Known etiological factor: gastroesophageal reflux.

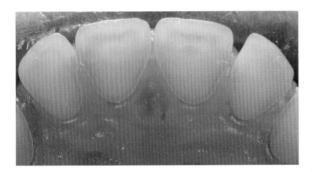

Fig. 9. Severe oral erosive tooth wear. Note the intact cervical enamel band and the pulp shining through. No endodontic complications or dental complaints. Age of patient: 29 years. Known etiological factor: Eating disorder (free from chronic vomiting for a couple of years).

forms of tooth wear, and criteria for the quantification of hard tissue loss. The size of the area affected is often given as the proportion of the affected to the sound tooth surface. The depth of a defect is estimated by using the criterion of dentine exposition. Thereby, a relation between exposed dentine and amount of substance loss is implicated. Most working groups have developed their own index modifications which had not yet reached broader use. Frequently used indices with particular regard to erosions are the indices used in the British Children's National Health and National Diet and Nutrition Surveys [13, 14] and the index suggested by Lussi [5] (table 2).

Two items included in the erosion indices are currently under discussion:

(1) The morphological criteria for occlusal/incisal surfaces are not strongly associated with erosive tissue loss. A study including subjects with substantially different nutrition patterns (an abrasive, an acidic, and an average western diet [15])

Table 1. Indices suggested by Smith and Knight [12] referring to tooth wear in general, and Eccles [11] including diagnostic criteria for erosive tooth wear

Score/class	Surface	Criteria
Tooth wear index according to Smith and Knight [12]		
0	B/L/O/I	No loss of enamel surface characteristics
	C	No loss of contour
1	B/L/O/I	Loss of enamel surface characteristics
	C	Minimal loss of contour
2	B/L/O	Loss of enamel exposing dentine for less than one-third of the surface
	I	Loss of enamel just exposing dentine
	C	Defect less than 1 mm deep
3	B/L/O	Loss of enamel exposing dentine for more than one-third of the surface
	I	Loss of enamel and substantial loss of dentine
	C	Defect less 1–2 mm deep
4	B/L/O	Complete loss of enamel, or pulp exposure, or exposure of secondary dentine
	I	Pulp exposure or exposure of secondary dentine
	C	Defect more than 2 mm deep, or pulp exposure, or exposure of secondary dentine
Index according to Eccles [11]		
Class I		Early stages of erosion, absence of developmental ridges, smooth, glazed surface occurring mainly on labial surfaces of maxillary incisors and canines
Class II	Facial	Dentine is involved for less than one-third of the surface Type 1: ovoid or crescentic, concave lesion at the cervical region of the surface, which should be differentiated from wedge-shaped lesions Type 2: irregular lesion entirely in the crown which has a punched-out appearance where the enamel is absent from the floor
Class IIIa	Facial	More extensive destruction of dentine particularly of the anterior teeth, most of the lesions affecting a large part of the surface, but some are localized and hollowed-out
Class IIIb	Lingual or palatal	Lesions of the surfaces for more than one third of their area, incisal edges become translucent due to loss of dentine, the dentine appears smooth, and in some cases is flat or hollowed-out, gingival and proximal margins have a white, etched appearance
Class IIIc	Incisal or occlusal	Incisal edges or occlusal surfaces are involved into dentine, flattening or cupping, restorations are seen raised above the surrounding tooth surface, incisal edges appear translucent due to undermined enamel
Class IIId	All	Severely affected teeth, where both labial and lingual surfaces are extensively involved

B = Buccal or lingual; C = cervical; I = incisal; L = lingual or palatal; O = occlusal.

Table 2. Frequently used erosion indices for the assessment of erosive tooth wear in children, adolescents and adults

Score	Surface	Criteria

Erosion index according to Lussi [5] (facial, lingual and occlusal surfaces of all teeth except third molars)

Facial

0		No erosion
		Surface with a smooth, silky-glazed appearance, absence of developmental ridges possible
1		Loss of surface enamel. Intact enamel found cervical to the lesion concavity in enamel, the width of which clearly exceeding its depth, thus, distinguishing it from toothbrush abrasion, undulating borders of the lesions are possible dentine is not involved
2		Involvement of dentine for less than one-half of the tooth surface
3		Involvement of dentine for more than one-half of the tooth surface

Occlusal/oral

0		No erosion
		Surface with a smooth, silky-glazed appearance
		Absence of developmental ridges possible
1		Slight erosion, rounded cusps, edges of restorations rising above the level of adjacent tooth surface, grooves on occlusal aspects
		Loss of surface enamel.
		Dentine is not involved
2		Severe erosion, more pronounced signs than grade 1
		Dentine is involved

Index used in the UK National Survey of Children's Dental Health (only facial and lingual surfaces of primary and permanent maxillary incisor teeth) and in the UK National Diet and Nutrition Surveys (additionally occlusal surfaces of the molar teeth)

Depth

0		Normal
1		Loss of surface characterization, enamel only – on incisor teeth there is loss of developmental ridges resulting in a smooth, glazed or 'ground glass' appearance
		On occlusal surfaces the cusps appear rounded and there may be depressions producing cupping
2		Enamel and dentine – loss of enamel exposing dentine. On incisors this may resemble a 'shoulder preparation' parallel to the crest of the gingivae, particularly on palatal surfaces
		The incisors may appear shorter and there may be chipping of the incisal edges
		On occlusal surfaces cupping and rounding-off of cusps is evident
		Restorations may be raised above the level of adjacent tooth surface
3		Enamel, dentine, and pulp – loss of enamel and dentine resulting in pulp exposure
9		Assessment cannot be made

Area

0		Normal
1		Less than one-third of surface involved
2		One-third to up to two-thirds of surface involved
3		More than two-thirds of surface involved
9		Assessment cannot be made

has clearly shown that the shape of occlusal/incisal lesions was similar in the abrasive and the acidic diet groups. During the process of breaking food, three-body abrasion can occur as result of the food bolus being moved between antagonistic teeth. In the early stage of chewing, when the food bolus separates the occlusal/incisal surfaces, the important feature is that the teeth do not mate and that this process tends to abrade the softer regions of the tooth surface resulting in a hollowing out of the dentine [16]. Significant occlusal tooth wear from mastication can occur either in the presence of high amounts of abrasives in the food bolus or in the case of acid-softening of enamel and dentine. This three-body abrasion would result in rounding and cupping of the cusps, and grooves on incisal edges making a differentiation between abrasion and erosion on occlusal surfaces difficult.

In contrast to the occlusal morphology, shallow defects on facial surfaces localized coronally from the enamel–cementum junction were common in the acidic diet group but were not observed in the abrasive diet group [15]. Consequently, flat-shaped defects occurring on smooth surfaces could be appraised as pathognomonic rather than the defects on the occlusal surfaces.

(2) The visual diagnosis of exposed dentine is difficult. Since changes in anatomical form, color or luster appeared to be easy to observe, the validity of this criterion still is not fully established.

In a recent study, teeth with signs of occlusal/incisal tooth wear of various etiology and severity were visually and histologically investigated regarding the presence of exposed dentine [17]. The study revealed two interesting findings. The first was that the accuracy (closeness of the visual decision to histological findings) was poor. Only 65% of areas with exposed dentine, 88% of areas with enamel present, and 67% of all areas examined were diagnosed correctly. The second finding was that exposed dentine was not related to significant amounts of tissue loss, a result that was also found in primary teeth [18]. Dentine was exposed in all cases of cupping or grooving even if only minor substance loss occurred. If cupping/grooving is assumed to be basically related to dentinal exposure, present grading of initial and advanced occlusal lesions should be reassessed.

Diagnosing exposed dentine, however, could be important for the therapeutic approach in cases of erosion or as a prognostic factor with respect to the progression rate.

Assessment of Progression Rate

The assessment of progression is important as it determines whether preventive measures taken were successful. Progression can be estimated by depth

[19–21], area [22], or volume [20]. Only little information is available about physiological wear rates. They were estimated to be annually 10–30 μm on occlusal [20, 23] and 7.5 μm on palatal surfaces [19]. The progression rate in patients with active erosive tissue loss could reach much higher rates [19].

Clinical signs for progression are a frosty appearance and absence of extrinsic staining. However, the quantitative assessment of tissue loss is difficult clinically as reference areas on the tooth surface might change over time. Consecutive study casts allow an estimation of wear progression [24] which might be sufficient in individual cases, but are neither sensitive nor suitable for exact quantification. Optical methods use microscopic techniques generating consecutive images of dental casts, which are superimposed [25, 26] and have significant errors. Surface mapping strategies aim to generate computerized superimposed 3D digital images by scanning consecutive dental casts profilometrically [20, 27], or with an optical 3D sensor [28], or by using electroconductive replicas [22]. The accuracy and the precision of these methods are suitable, but mostly expensive equipment is needed. A relatively practicable procedure was suggested from Bartlett et al. [19], which was further modified by Schlueter et al. [21]. Metal markers were applied on tooth surfaces serving as reference and identification area for profilometric measurements. The procedure appears somewhat less sensitive compared to elaborate surface mapping, but is applicable without extensive equipment. Other applications are discussed in the chapter 10 by Attin, this vol, pp 152–172.

Even if attempts have been made to introduce methods for the assessment of progression rates, there is still need for thoroughly evaluated, sensitive, practicable and preferably chairside procedures.

Future Perspectives

Four major points regarding the diagnosis of erosive tooth wear appear important for future activities:
- There is need for standardization of terminology and indices.
- Items of currently used indices should be reconsidered with respect to the validity of diagnostic criteria (particularly for occlusal surfaces) and grading (the relevance and diagnosis of exposed dentine).
- Considerations about the differentiation between pathological and physiological erosive tooth wear (on an individual level as well as in the frame of epidemiological research), which, inter alia, is a matter of age and progression rate are necessary.
- The development of practicable and preferably chairside diagnostic tools for progression rate is needed.

References

1   Kidd EAM, Mejàre I, Nyvad B: Clinical and radiographic diagnosis; in Fejerskov O, Kidd EAM (eds): Dental Caries: The Disease and Its Clinical Management. Copenhagen, Blackwell Munksgaard, 2003, pp 111–128.

2   Bartlett D: The implication of laboratory research on tooth wear and erosion. Oral Dis 2005;11:3–6.

3   Lussi A, Jaeggi T, Zero D: The role of diet in the aetiology of dental erosion. Caries Res 2004;38 (suppl):34–44.

4   Linkosalo E, Markkanen H: Dental erosions in relation to lactovegetarian diet. Scand J Dent Res 1985;93:436–441.

5   Lussi A: Dental erosion clinical diagnosis and case history taking. Eur J Oral Sci 1996;104:191–198.

6   Larsen IB, Westergaard J, Stoltze K, Gyntelberg F, Holmstrup P: A clinical index for evaluating and monitoring dental erosion. Community Dent Oral Epidemiol 2000;28:211–217.

7   O'Sullivan EA: A new index for the measurement of erosion in children. Eur J Paediatr Dent 2000;1:69–74.

8   Al-Malik MI, Holt RD, Bedi R: Erosion, caries and rampant caries in preschool children in Jeddah, Saudi Arabia. Community Dent Oral Epidemiol 2002;30:16–23.

9   Arnadottir IB, Saemundsson SR, Holbrook WP: Dental erosion in Icelandic teenagers in relation to dietary and lifestyle factors. Acta Odontol Scand 2003;61:25–28.

10 Harding MA, Whelton H, O'Mullane DM, Cronin M: Dental erosion in 5-year-old Irish school children and associated factors: a pilot study. Community Dent Health 2003;20:165–170.

11 Eccles JD: Dental erosion of nonindustrial origin. A clinical survey and classification. J Prosthet Dent 1979;42:649–653.

12 Smith BG, Knight JK: An index for measuring the wear of teeth. Br Dent J 1984;156:435–438.

13 O'Brian M: Children's Dental Health in the United Kingdom 1993. Office of Population Censuses and Surveys 1994. London, Her Majesty's Stationary Office, 1993.

14 Nunn JH, Gordon PH, Morris AJ, Pine CM, Walker A: Dental erosion – changing prevalence? A review of British National childrens' surveys. Int J Paediatr Dent 2003;13:98–105.

15 Ganss C, Klimek J, Borkowski N: Characteristics of tooth wear in relation to different nutritional patterns including contemporary and medieval subjects. Eur J Oral Sci 2002;110:54–60.

16 Mair LH: Wear in the mouth: the tribological dimension; in Addy M, Embery G, Edgar WM, Orchardson R (eds): Tooth Wear and Sensitivity: Clinical Advances in Restorative Dentistry. London, Martin Dunitz, 2000, pp 181–188.

17 Ganss C, Klimek J, Lussi A: Accuracy and consistency of the visual diagnosis of exposed dentine on worn occlusal/incisal surfaces. Caries Res 2005;40:208–212.

18 Al-Malik MI, Holt RD, Bedi R, Speight PM: Investigation of an index to measure tooth wear in primary teeth. J Dent 2001;29:103–107.

19 Bartlett DW, Blunt L, Smith BG: Measurement of tooth wear in patients with palatal erosion. Br Dent J 1997;182:179–184.

20 Pintado MR, Anderson GC, DeLong R, Douglas WH: Variation in tooth wear in young adults over a two-year period. J Prosthet Dent 1997;77:313–320.

21 Schlueter N, Ganss C, De Sanctis S, Klimek J: Evaluation of a profilometrical method for monitoring erosive tooth wear. Eur J Oral Sci 2005;113:505–511.

22 Chadwick RG, Mitchell HL: Conduct of an algorithm in quantifying simulated palatal surface tooth erosion. J Oral Rehabil 2001;28:450–456.

23 Lambrechts P, Braem M, Vuylsteke-Wauters M, Vanherle G: Quantitative in vivo wear of human enamel. J Dent Res 1989;68:1752–1754.

24 Öhrn R, Angmar-Månsson B: Oral status of 35 subjects with eating disorders – a 1-year study. Eur J Oral Sci 2000;108:275–280.

25 Sorvari R, Kiviranta I: A semiquantitative method of recording experimental tooth erosion and estimation occlusal wear in the rat. Arch Oral Biol 1988;33:217–220.

26 Mistry M, Grenby TH: Erosion by soft drinks of rat molar teeth assessed by digital image analysis. Caries Res 1993;27:21–25.

27   Pesun IJ, Olson AK, Hodges JS, Anderson GC: In vivo evaluation of the surface of posterior resin composite restorations: a pilot study. J Prosthet Dent 2000;84:353–359.

28   Mehl A, Gloger W, Kunzelmann KH, Hickel R: A new optical 3-D device for the detection of wear. J Dent Res 1997;76:1799–1807.

Priv.-Doz. Dr. Carolina Ganss
Department of Conservative and Preventive Dentistry
Dental Clinic, Justus Liebig University Giessen
Schlangenzahl 14
DE–35392 Giessen (Germany)

Lussi A (ed): Dental Erosion.
Monogr Oral Sci. Basel, Karger, 2006, vol 20, pp 44–65

....

Prevalence, Incidence and Distribution of Erosion

Thomas Jaeggi, Adrian Lussi

Department of Preventive, Restorative and Pediatric Dentistry,
School of Dental Medicine, University of Bern, Bern, Switzerland

Abstract

There is some evidence that the presence of erosion is growing steadily. Because of different scoring systems, samples and examiners, it is difficult to compare and judge the outcome of the studies. Preschool children aged between 2 and 5 years showed erosion on deciduous teeth in 6–50% of the subjects. Young schoolchildren (aged 5–9) already had erosive lesions on permanent teeth in 14% of the cases. In the adolescent group (aged between 9 and 17) 11–100% of the young people examined showed signs of erosion. Incidence data (= increase of subjects with erosion) evaluated in three of these studies were 12% over 2 years, 18% over 5 years and 27% over 1.5 years. In adults (aged between 18 and 88), prevalence data ranged between 4 and 82%. Incidence data are scarce; only one study was found and this showed an incidence of 5% for the younger and 18% for the older examined group (= increase of tooth surfaces with erosion). Prevalence data indicated that males had somewhat more erosive tooth wear than females. The distribution of erosion showed a predominance of occlusal surfaces (especially mandibular first molars), followed by facial surfaces (anterior maxillary teeth). Oral erosion was frequently found on maxillary incisors and canines. Overall, prevalence data are not homogeneous. Nevertheless, there is already a trend for more pronounced rate of erosion in younger age groups. Therefore, it is important to detect at-risk patients early to initiate adequate preventive measures.

Erosive tooth wear is a common condition in developed societies. The lesions are often found independent of the age of the population examined. It is difficult to compare the results of epidemiological studies because of different examination standards used (calibration of examiner(s), scoring system, number and site of teeth) and different nonhomogeneous groups examined (age, gender, number of examined individuals, geographical location). It is easier to recruit schoolchildren for clinical examinations than adults. Therefore, more studies on children and adolescents than on adults are found. Nevertheless, it is important to record erosive tooth lesions to gather data about the prevalence, the distribution and the incidence of erosion.

If we want to understand the occurrence and distribution of erosive lesions, we have to be aware of the different etiological factors, such as reflux, vomiting and diet [1–7]. These causes are discussed in other chapters.

Susceptibility to Erosive Tooth Wear in Children and Adults

There are some differences in the anatomical structure of deciduous teeth compared with permanent teeth. The enamel of the deciduous teeth is less thick than the enamel of the permanent dentition. Therefore, the erosive process reaches the dentine earlier leading to more advanced lesions developing following an exposure to acids. Currently, there is contradictory evidence to state that deciduous teeth are more susceptible to dental erosion than permanent teeth [8–12] (see chapter 9 by Lussi et al., this vol, pp 140–151). The mechanical resistance of deciduous enamel is lower than that of permanent teeth because of the reduced hardness of it [13]. Therefore, substance loss in deciduous teeth can be more pronounced following erosive tooth wear than in permanent teeth. Conversely, functional and parafunctional forces in children are, in general, less than those found in adults. In summary, the differences in susceptibility to erosive tooth wear between children and adults seem to be small.

Prevalence, Incidence and Distribution of Erosion in Children and Adolescents

Dental Erosion in Preschool Children and Young Schoolchildren
Clinical Studies with Partial Recording of the Teeth
A study of 987 children that were aged between 2 and 5 years from 17 kindergarten schools showed that 309 (31%) had evidence of erosion and 123 (13%) of them showed involvement of dentine and/or pulp. The measurement of the erosion was confined to primary maxillary incisors [14]. Another dental examination was carried out on 1,949 children aged 3–5 years in China, and a total of 112 children (5.7%) showed erosion on their primary maxillary incisors. Ninety-five (4.9%) were judged to have erosion confined to enamel and 17 (0.9%) were scored as having erosion extending into dentine or pulp. A significantly higher prevalence of erosion was observed in children who had frequently consumed fruit drinks as a baby and whose parents had a higher education level [15]. Harding et al. [16] found a link between low socioeconomic

status, frequent consumption of fruit squash and carbonated drinks and the occurrence of dental erosion. In this sample, 47% of 202 5-year-old children showed dental erosion, with 21% of lesions in an advanced state (erosion affecting the dentine or pulp). Only palatal and labial surfaces of primary maxillary teeth were assessed.

Clinical Studies with Full Mouth Recording

Millward et al. [17] examined a total of 178 4-year-old children and found that almost the half of them showed signs of erosion. Frequently, the palatal surfaces of the maxillary incisors were affected with lesions reaching the dentine. The authors investigated socioeconomic group and found a greater prevalence of dental erosion in the higher socioeconomic groups.

The prevalence, severity and distribution of erosive lesions in children living in rural Switzerland were investigated. A total of 42 children, were examined, aged between 5 and 9 years. All children had one or more erosive lesions confined to enamel on the occlusal surface and 48% of them showed at least one lesion extending into dentine. Fourteen percent of the children had one or more erosive lesions detected on the occlusal surfaces of permanent teeth. Facial and oral erosions were scarce and involved deciduous teeth only. Ten percent had lesions on facial surfaces and 7% on palatal surfaces; all were confined to enamel. Erosion extending into dentine occurred on the facial surfaces in 5% of the children and on the palatal surfaces in 2%. The facial erosive lesions were mostly located on the primary central incisors. The most commonly affected tooth surfaces were the occlusal surfaces of the deciduous molars. Oral erosions were seldom found on the permanent maxillary incisors [18].

Dental Erosion in Adolescents

Study with Assessment of Models

Ganss et al. [19] examined a large sample of preorthodontic study models of adolescents (1,000 individuals, mean age 11.4 ± 3.3 years); they included all surfaces of primary teeth. Moderate erosive lesions were found in 70.6% (facial/oral surfaces: shallow concavities less than one-third of the surface; occlusal surfaces: small pits and slightly rounded cusps, moderate cupping) and advanced erosion in 26.4% of the children (facial/oral surfaces: deeper or more extended concavities [more than one-third]; occlusal surfaces: severe cupping and grooving). The majority of lesions were found on the occlusal or incisal surfaces (molars and canines). In the permanent dentition, 11.6% of the individuals had at least one tooth with moderate erosion and 0.2% with advanced erosion. The most affected teeth were the first molars in the mandibular jaw. After a period of 5 years, 265 of the children were followed up by examination of their final study models. Longitudinal observation revealed that subjects with erosive lesions in their deciduous dentition had a significantly increased risk (relative risk 3.9) for development of erosion in their permanent dentition. The incidence of erosion for permanent teeth was as follows: individuals with at least one tooth with moderate erosion had an increased risk from 5.3 to 23%; those with advanced erosion this risk was from 0.4 to 1.5%.

Clinical Studies with Partial Recording of the Teeth

Truin et al. [20] evaluated the prevalence of erosive wear among 12-year-old children in The Hague, the Netherlands. The examination was limited to the palatal surfaces of incisors and canines, and the occlusal surfaces of first molars in the permanent dentition. Twenty-four percent of the 12-year-olds exhibited signs of erosion. Erosive wear was only found on first molars in 11% of the children and 9% of them also had a maxillary front tooth affected. No significant differences were found between the prevalence of erosion and the different socioeconomic-status groups examined. However, more boys (28%) than girls (18%) had erosion in any form. Examination of the incisors and molars of 1,753 12-year-old children showed a prevalence of tooth erosion of 59.7%, with 2.7% exhibiting exposed dentine [21]. Significantly more erosion was detected in boys than girls. In addition, those with caries experience were found to have more erosion, as were more Caucasians compared with those of Asian origin. Socio-economically advantaged Caucasian children had significantly less tooth erosion than the other examined groups. The culture of the children examined appeared to influence the prevalence of erosion. The distribution of erosive lesions was as follows: Erosion occurred most frequently on the palatal surfaces of maxillary incisors (49%) and maxillary molars (53%), as well as the buccal surfaces of mandibular molars (50%). Dentine was exposed to the greatest extent on the occlusal surfaces of mandibular molars (2.2%). Tooth erosion was symmetrical around the midline [21]. The same authors re-examined 1,308 children of the same sample 2 years later, and found an incidence of erosion of 12.3%. One hundred and sixty-one children who had no evidence of erosion at 12 years developed erosion over the subsequent 2 years. Erosion was present in 56.3% of 12-year-olds and in 64.1% by the age of 14. The proportion of subjects with exposure of deep enamel increased from 4.9 to 13.1%, and those with involved dentine from 2.4 to 8.7%. Boys showed significantly more erosion than girls at both ages, as did Caucasian compared to Asian children in both age groups [22]. Convenience samples of 129 children (aged 11–13 years) in the USA and 125 children in the UK were examined, only the palatal and facial surfaces of the maxillary incisors were assessed. Prevalence data were as follows: 41% of the US and 37% of the UK children showed dental erosion. The lesions were mostly confined to enamel [23]. Chadwick et al. [24] measured the prevalence of palatal erosion of the central maxillary incisors of 197 schoolchildren (aged 11–13 years) with a replica technique. They found 58.5% low erosions (none to limited, normal wear), 28.7% moderate erosions (obvious change in anatomical form but no need for treatment) and 12.3% severe erosions (marked change in anatomical form and need for treatment). Each subject was recorded at baseline and after 9 and 18 months. They concluded that evidence of previous palatal erosion did not predict future erosion. In London, a cross-section design study containing 525 14-year-old schoolchildren showed a prevalence of 16.9% for facial and 12% for palatal surface erosion (only the maxillary incisors were examined) [25]. In the North-West of England a total of 2,385 14-year-old children (48% male, 52% female) were examined for tooth wear. A total of 1,276 children (53%) had at least one tooth surface (mean 2 surfaces) with exposed dentine. Significantly more males had dentine exposed than females. Incisal or occlusal wear into dentine was seen most frequently on central incisors and mandibular first molars (tooth wear was scored on all surfaces of the maxillary six and mandibular six anterior teeth and on the occlusal surfaces of the first molars) [26].

Clinical Studies with Full Mouth Recording

Caglar et al. [27] in a sample of 153 schoolchildren (aged 11 years) in Istanbul, Turkey, investigated the occurrence of erosive defects. Twenty-eight percent of them exhibited dental erosion but no relationship was found between erosion and possible related sources. A longitudinal study of dental erosion in 73 12-year old girls showed the following: 68% had dental erosion at the beginning of the investigation. After 1.5 years 65 girls were re-examined, and 95% showed the clinical appearance of erosive lesions. Therefore, the incidence was 27%. The mean number of teeth affected was 2.2 at the start of the investigation and 5.6 after 18 months [28]. Milosevic et al. [29] examined a total of 1,035 children (mean age: 14 years) in 10 schools in Liverpool, UK. Thirty percent of them had tooth wear lesions with involvement of dentine, mainly incisally. Eight percent also exhibited exposed dentine on occlusal and/or palatal surfaces; mainly the occlusal surfaces of the first mandibular molars and the palatal aspects of the maxillary incisors were affected. Statistical evaluation showed significantly more erosion in males than in females. Al-Dlaigan et al. [30] established the prevalence of erosion in a cluster random sample of 418 14-year-old teenagers (209 girls, 209 boys) in Birmingham, UK. They found that 48% of the children had erosion within enamel, 51% had erosion within enamel, possibly with slight involvement of dentine and 1% had erosion with advanced involvement of dentine. They postulated a relationship between low socioeconomic status and the occurrence of erosion. The majority of tooth surfaces showed evidence of enamel erosion on both maxillary and mandibular teeth on the facial and oral aspects. Defects with visible dentine involvement were mainly found on the incisal edges of most anterior teeth, whereas dentinal erosions were most common on the maxillary and mandibular facial surfaces of anterior teeth. Significantly more males than females showed these lesions. In Reykjavik, Iceland, 20% of a cohort sample of 15-year-olds was examined (n = 278). The investigators found that a total of 21.6% of the subjects suffered from dental erosion, two thirds of these were male. Enamel erosion was found in 72% of the cases, 23% showed dentinal erosion and 5% had severe dentinal erosion [31]. Van Rijkom et al. [33] investigated the prevalence and distribution of smooth-bordered tooth wear in teenagers in The Hague, the Netherlands. A sample of 345 10–13-year-olds and 400 15- and 16-year-olds were examined clinically. The investigation was based on a modification of the index of Lussi et al. [32]. In the younger age group, 3% of the subjects showed visible smooth wear on enamel. Only one subject (0.3%) had deep smooth enamel wear. In the older age group, 30% of the subjects had visible smooth wear of enamel, in 11% deep smooth wear of enamel and in one case smooth wear into dentine was found. In the majority of subjects, first molars and maxillary anterior teeth were affected. The prevalence of visible smooth wear was significantly higher in boys than in girls and it tended to increase with increasing socioeconomic status [33]. To describe the prevalence of eroded tooth surfaces among 15–17-year-old schoolchildren in a Danish city, 558 subjects were examined for dental erosions. It was found that 14% of the children had more than three surfaces affected; the palatal surfaces more so than the facial surfaces. No evidence of lesions in dentine was observed [34].

Reviewing the data from the national dental surveys of young people in the UK, a trend towards a higher prevalence of erosion in children aged between 3.5 and 4.5 years was found. Overall, the prevalence data from cross-sectional national studies indicated that erosion increased with age of children and adolescents over time. In addition, dietary habits, the presence or absence of gastroesophageal reflux and sociodemographic parameters had some influence on dental erosion [35].

A survey of the localization of erosion in children and adolescents is given in table 1. Prevalence and incidence data are listed in table 2.

To summarize, the results from several epidemiological studies involving erosive tooth wear in children and adolescents, the following conclusions can be drawn: with increasing mean age of the population-group examined, there is a trend to more erosive lesions detected. Males seem to develop more erosion than females. This involves the palatal surface of the maxillary incisors and the occlusal surface of the mandibular first molars. The relationship between the presence of erosive lesions and the socioeconomic status of the population-groups investigated is controversial and no consensus has been agreed.

Table 1. Localization of erosion in children and adolescents: a survey of different epidemiological studies listed in the order of the age of the examined samples

Author(s)	Year	Age (years)	Localization
Millward et al. [17]	1994	4	Primary dentition: palatal surfaces of the maxillary incisors
Jaeggi and Lussi [18]	2004	5–9	Primary dentition: occlusal surfaces of all teeth (predominantly molars); facial and oral surfaces of the maxillary incisors (scarce) Permanent dentition: occlusal surfaces of the first molars
Ganss et al. [19]	2001	8–14	Primary dentition: occlusal (incisal) surfaces of molars and canines Permanent dentition: occlusal surfaces of mandibular first molars
Milosevic et al. [29]	1994	14	Palatal and incisal surfaces of maxillary incisors; occlusal surfaces of the first mandibular molars
Al-Dlaigan et al. [30]	2001	14	Low erosion: majority of tooth surfaces; moderate erosion: incisal edges of anterior teeth; sever erosion: maxillary and mandibular facial surfaces of anterior teeth
Van Rijkom et al. [33]	2002	10–13 15–16	First molars and maxillary anterior teeth
Larsen et al. [34]	2005	15–17	Palatal surfaces of maxillary incisors

Prevalence, Incidence and Distribution of Erosion in Adults

Studies with Assessment of Extracted Teeth or Models

As early as 1972, Sognnaes et al. [36] found in a sample of 10,827 extracted teeth 18% with signs of erosion-like lesions. They noted that mandibular teeth had a higher frequency of such lesions than the corresponding maxillary teeth (21% compared to 13%). The highest percentage of erosion-like lesions was found in mandibular incisors (28%). Khan et al. [37], in a cross-sectional study, investigated the presence, absence and relative size of cupped lesions on cusps and occlusal fissures of premolar and permanent molar teeth using image analysis of study models. The frequencies of the following five types of lesions on the tooth sites were scored as follows: unaffected (46%), small (17%), medium (8%), large cuspal-cupped lesions (4%), and fissure involvement by cupping (3%). Twenty-two percent of the possible tooth sites were absent. The influence of age was evaluated by comparison of the models of 59 younger (aged 13–27) and 57 older subjects (aged 28–70). They found a linear increase in lesion number and size with age. Cupped lesions often occurred on mandibular first molar cusp tips, and attained greater extension in adults under 27 years compared with older subjects. They concluded that the

Table 2. Prevalence and incidence of erosion in children and adolescents (% of examined subjects): a survey of different epidemiological studies listed in the order of the age of the examined samples

Author(s)	Year	Sample		examination	Erosion prevalence	Erosion incidence	Conclusion
		Age (years)	n				
Al-Malik et al. [14]	2002	2–5	987	Clinical	31%	–	1/3 with erosion, and 1/3 to 1/2 of them showed involvement of dentine or pulp
Luo et al. [15]	2005	3–5	1,949	Clinical	5.7%	–	4.9% with erosion confined to enamel, 0.9% with involvement of dentine or pulp
Millward et al. [17]	1994	4	178	Clinical	50%	–	Almost half of the examined children showed erosion
Harding et al. [16]	2003	5	202	Clinical	47%	–	21% of the erosive lesions with involvement of dentine or pulp
Jaeggi and Lussi [18]	2004	5–9	42	Clinical	100%/14.3%	–	100% of the children with enamel erosion, 47.6% with dentinal erosion, 14.3% already with erosion on permanent teeth
Caglar et al. [27]	2005	11	153	Clinical	28%	–	No significant differences in prevalence data between girls and boys
Ganss et al. [19]	2001	8–14	1,000	Models	70.6%/11.6%	–	Primary teeth: 70.6% with moderate erosion, 26.4% with advanced erosion; permanent teeth: 11.6% (moderate erosion) and 0.2% (advanced erosion)
		16	265	Models	–/23%	–/18% within 5 years	Permanent teeth (longitudinally): increase of erosion from 5.3 to 23% (moderate erosion) and from 0.4 to 1.5% (advanced erosion)
Dugmore and Rock [21]	2004	12	1,753	Clinical	59.7%	–	2.7% of the erosive lesions with involvement of dentine
Truin et al. [20]	2005	12	324	Clinical	24%	–	24% of the children showed signs of erosion
Deery et al. [23]	2000	11–13	129 (US) 125 (UK)	Clinical	41% (US) 37% (UK)	–	Erosion was mostly confined to enamel

Table 2. (continued)

Author(s)	Year	Sample Age (years)	n	examination	Erosion prevalence	Erosion incidence	Conclusion
Chadwick et al. [24]	2005	11–13	197	Clinical (replica technique)	100%	–	58.5% with low erosion, 28.7% with moderate erosion, 12.3% with severe erosion
Nunn et al. [28]	2001	12/13.5	73/65	Clinical	68%/95%	27% after 1.5 years	Mean number of affected teeth rose from 2.2 to 5.6
Dugmore and Rock [22]	2003	12/14	1,308	Clinical	56.3%/64.1%	12.3% within two years	Deep enamel erosions increased from 4.9 to 13.1% and with dentine involvement from 2.4 to 8.7%
Milosevic et al. [29]	1994	14	1,035	Clinical	30%	–	30% with involvement of dentine; more males than females showed tooth wear lesions
Williams et al. [25]	1999	14	525	Clinical	17%[a]/12%[a]	–	17% of facial and 12% of palatal surfaces of maxillary incisors with erosion
Al-Dlaigan et al. [30]	2001	14	418	Clinical	100%	–	48% with low erosion, 51% with moderate erosion, 1% with severe erosion
Bardsley et al. [26]	2004	14	2,385	Clinical	53%	–	53% had at least one tooth with exposed dentine
Arnadottir et al. [31]	2003	15	278	Clinical	21.6%	–	72% of the erosions confined to enamel, 23% reaching the dentine, 5% reaching deep into dentine
Van Rijkom et al. [33]	2002	10–13 / 15–16	345 / 400	Clinical	3% / 30%/11%	–	3% of the younger and 30% of the older age group showed visible smooth wear; 11% of the older age group had deep enamel lesions
Larsen et al. [34]	2005	15–17	558	Clinical	14%	–	14% more than 3 surfaces of erosion

[a] % of examined tooth surfaces.

mandibular first permanent molar is an indicator for the age of onset and severity of dental erosion.

Studies with Partial Recording of the Teeth

Xhonga et al. [38] investigated the progression of erosive tooth wear in 14 patients with erosion-like patterns (aged between 26 and 65 years). They found an average daily rate of progression of approximately 1 μm. In another study, a random selection of 95 males with a mean age of 20.9 years was scored. Only the maxillary anterior teeth were included. They concluded that 28% of the teeth in this sample showed pronounced dental erosion [39].

Clinical Studies with Full Mouth Recording

In a two-centre study, Xhonga and Valdmanis [40] examined a total of 527 randomly selected patients for erosive tooth wear (aged 14–88 years). Erosion-like lesions found were divided into three groups: minor, moderate and severe. This study suggested that the prevalence in the USA was about 25% for erosive tooth wear. Minor lesions (prevalence about 20%) were found most often in premolar and anterior teeth. Moderate lesions were scarce (prevalence about 4%) and equally distributed. Severe lesions (prevalence about 25%) were found predominantly in molar regions, followed by premolars. In a case-control study, in the Metropolitan Helsinki area, Finland, 100 controls (mean age: 36.3 years; range: 17–83 years) were randomly selected by dentists. Five of these control subjects had erosion. Therefore, the prevalence of dental erosion in patients of this area was 5%. Although only 5 of the examined individuals showed erosive defects, most of them admitted to having regular exposure to acid. Dietary exposure was present in 21, gastric exposure in 19 and both exposure types in 5 cases. Fifty-five of the controls did not exceed any of the exposure limits [2]. Jaeggi et al. [41] assessed a sample of 417 Swiss army recruits (aged between 19 and 25 years). Clinical examination showed dental erosions on all tooth surfaces with the most pronounced defects found on occlusal aspects. Eighty-two percent of the screened recruits had erosive lesions within enamel on these tooth surfaces. Occlusal lesions with involvement of dentine were found in 128 recruits (30.7%). Facial defects occurred in 60 cases (14.4%, enamel erosion) and 2 cases (0.5%, dentinal erosion). Palatal erosions were scarce with only 3 (0.7%) individuals affected. The localization of the erosive lesions were as follows: facial erosions were frequent on canines and premolars of both jaws, occlusal erosions on first molars and premolars of both jaws and palatal erosions on maxillary anterior teeth. Lussi et al. [32] examined the frequency and severity of erosion on all tooth surfaces of 391 randomly selected persons from two age groups: 26–30 and 46–50 years. Erosions confined to enamel were found on facial surfaces in 11.9% of the younger and 9.6% of the older subjects. Whereas, more pronounced erosive

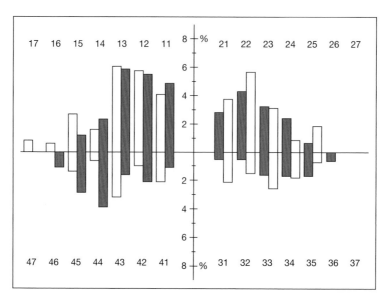

Fig. 1. Distribution of erosion confined to enamel on facial surfaces of two age groups (dark columns = 26–30 years; white columns = 46–50 years; n = 391) [32].

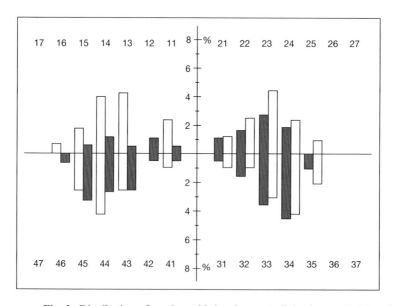

Fig. 2. Distribution of erosion with involvement of dentine on facial surfaces of two age groups (dark columns = 26–30 years; white columns = 46–50 years; n = 391) [32].

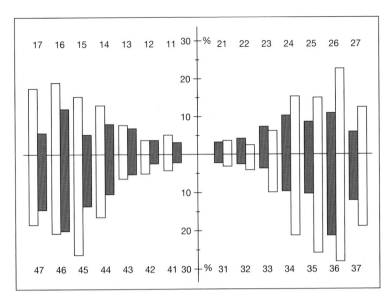

Fig. 3. Distribution of erosion confined to enamel on occlusal surfaces of two age groups (dark columns = 26–30 years; white columns = 46–50 years; n = 391) [32].

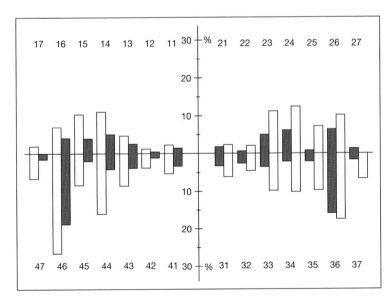

Fig. 4. Distribution of erosion with involvement of dentine on occlusal surfaces of two age groups (dark columns = 26–30 years; white columns = 46–50 years; n = 391) [32].

defects (erosion with involvement of dentine) were found in 7.7% of the younger and 13.2% of the older age group. On average, 3.5 teeth per person in the younger and 2.8 teeth per person in the older age group were affected. Occlusally, erosions confined to enamel were found in 35.6% of the younger and 40.1% of the older persons. At least one severe erosive lesion was observed in 29.9% of the younger and 42.6% of the older sample. Therefore, 3.2 teeth per person in the younger and 3.9 teeth per person in the older group showed these advanced lesions. Statistical analyses revealed a significant impact of the consumption of erosive drinks and foodstuffs on facial and occlusal erosions. On the palatal surfaces in 3.6% of the younger and 6.1% of the older examined individuals slight erosive defects were found (erosion confined to enamel). Severe palatal erosions were scarce and highly associated with chronic vomiting (figs. 1–4). To determine the progression of erosive defects, the same authors re-examined 55 persons 6 years later. They found a distinct progression of erosion on facial and occlusal surfaces. The increase in the defects was more pronounced in the older age group. The prevalence of occlusal erosions involving dentine rose from 3 to 8% (younger age group) and from 8 to 26% (older age group). An increase in facial erosions was observed over the entire dentition but especially in premolar and molar areas. The increase in erosion with denudation of dentine ranged from 4.2% (tooth 16) to 17.6% (tooth 15) with no differences between maxillary and mandibular jaws. The increase in occlusal lesions in the premolar and molar areas was even more marked: for dentinal erosion from 0.1% (tooth 35) to 33.4% (tooth 14), again with no differences between maxillary and mandibular jaws. Oral erosions were detected only in the maxillary jaw. The most marked increase in oral erosion was found in the central incisors (from 6 to 10%). Although all patients initially were personally informed about the risk factors for the development and progression of erosive lesions, they did not change their nutritional habits. Statistical analyses showed that 28% of the variability of the progression of erosion could be explained with the consumption of nutritional acids and age. Further, it was shown that one-third of the patients accounted for about two-thirds of the total progression. Four or more nutritional acidic intakes per day were associated with higher progression when it was combined with low buffer capacity of stimulated saliva and hard toothbrushes (p < 0.01) [42] (figs. 5, 6). Schiffner et al. [43] investigated in a nationwide representative study in Germany, the prevalence of noncarious cervical lesions involving two age groups: 35–44 and 65–74 years. They found that 42.1% of the younger and 46.3% of the older individuals showed at least one of these lesions (mean number of lesions per subject for the two groups: 2.2 and 2.5 teeth, respectively). Erosion confined to enamel was found in 6.4% of the younger and 4.1% of the older age group. Advanced erosion with involvement of dentine was present in 4.3% of the younger and 3.8% of the older individuals. Cervical wedge shaped defects were found in 31.5% of the younger

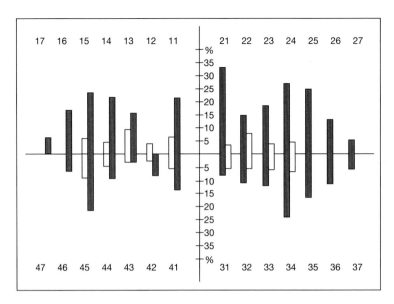

Fig. 5. Progression of erosion on facial surfaces (46–50 years group): Distribution of all the defects – if present – at baseline (light columns) and 6 years later (dark columns) [modified from 42].

and 35% of the older population group. There was a significantly higher prevalence of noncarious cervical lesions in men than in women. Considering the reduced number of teeth, a significant increase in the presence of these alterations was found in older subjects.

Clinical Studies of Specific Population Groups

Mathew et al. [44] examined the erosion status of 304 athletes from the Ohio State University, USA. The athletes ranged in age from 18 to 28 years. Total prevalence of dental erosion of this specific population was 36.5%, of which 2.3% represented facial erosion, 35.5% occlusal erosion, and 0.7% palatal erosion. Enamel erosion was detected in 75.2% of the cases, the remaining showed dentinal involvement as well. The mandibular first permanent molar was the most often affected tooth, especially the occlusal surface of this tooth. No relationship was found between consumption of sports drinks and dental erosion. In another study, Ganss et al. [45] examined the frequency and severity of dental erosion and its association with nutritional and oral hygiene factors in subjects living on a raw food diet. As part of a larger investigation, 130 subjects whose ingestion of raw food was more than 95% of the total food intake were examined (age of subjects

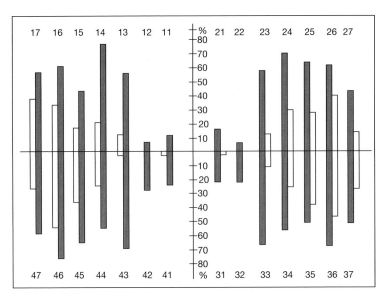

Fig. 6. Progression of erosion on occlusal surfaces (46–50 years group): Distribution of all the defects – if present – at baseline (light columns) and 6 years later (dark columns) [modified from 42].

was 18–63 years; median duration of the diet: 39 months). Dental erosion was measured using study models. The results were compared with those of 76 sex- and age-matched, randomly selected controls. Compared to the control group, subjects living on a raw food diet had significantly more dental erosion: at least one tooth with severe erosion was found in 60.5% (controls: 31.6%), moderate erosion in 37.2% (controls: 55.2%) and only 2.3% (controls: 13.2%) of the subjects had no erosive defects. In both groups (raw food and controls), the risk of erosive lesions was highest on occlusal surfaces. On these surfaces, erosive defects were distributed evenly but pronounced at mandibular first molars (raw food group only). Facial erosion was most frequently detected in the anterior region of the maxilla, and in canines and premolars in the mandible. On palatal surfaces, erosion was found in the maxillary and mandibular anterior area. Tuominen et al. [46] investigating dental erosion in a population from a factory found an average prevalence of erosion for the control group of 26%.

Tooth Wear Studies in Context with Erosion

As already discussed, not only erosion per se leads to tooth surface loss. The degradation of tooth surface occurs mainly because of chemical and/or mechanical influences. The damage of dental hard substance increases dramatically if acid etched surfaces are mechanical loaded [6]. For the clinical evaluation of tooth wear, it is also important to take the age of the patient into consideration. Obviously, it is more common for older people to show more tooth-substance loss than younger people [42]. Smith and Knight [47] defined an index, which considers the relationship between age and the damage to teeth caused by erosion, attrition, abrasion and combinations of these conditions (see chapter 2 by Ganss, this vol, pp 9–16). They proposed threshold levels to distinguish physiological and pathological levels of tooth wear: the six age groups were: 25 years or less; the four decades from 26 to 65 years; and 66 years and over. The threshold levels were adjusted following the results obtained from different studies. The index showed good reproducibility: 70–93% with seven trained examiners. In order to enhance its effectiveness the tooth wear index of Smith and Knight was modified [48]. A study in South East England investigated the prevalence of tooth wear in 1,007 dental patients. More than 93,500 tooth surfaces were examined and over all 5.1% had wear which exceeded the threshold values. Only 9 patients had completely unworn dentitions. The 15–26-year age group showed 5.73% of tooth surfaces which where worn to an unacceptable degree; the three intermediate groups (age groups 26–35, 36–45 and 46–55 years) had values between 3.37 and 4.62%, the 56–65-year age group had 8.19%, and the over 65-year age group had 8.84% of the surfaces with pathological tooth wear. In particular, the older age groups had higher levels of unacceptable tooth wear, and men tended to have slightly more wear than women [49]. From the Community of Jönköping (Sweden), 585 randomly selected dentate individuals were screened for occlusal and incisal tooth wear. The age of the people examined was 20–80 years. The results showed an increase of severity and prevalence of wear with age. Men presented with more teeth showing occlusal wear than women. The factors significantly related to tooth wear were: number of teeth present; age; sex; occurrence of bruxism; use of snuff, and saliva buffer capacity [50]. The tooth wear index of a random sample of adults aged 45 years and over from Newcastle-upon-Tyne (UK) was assessed by Donachie and Walls [51]. Five hundred and eighty-six subjects were dentate and able to undergo the examinations. Results showed significantly increasing wear levels with increasing age for all cervical and occlusal/incisal tooth surfaces. Especially in the older age cohort, occlusal/incisal surfaces showed some of the highest mean wear scores. With the exception of palatal surfaces of maxillary anterior teeth, no significant variation in tooth wear with age was found for buccal or palatal surfaces. The mean wear scores were greater in males than females. Only a small variation was found between subjects of different social classes. As already discussed, some of the citied investigations only used a partial recording score system, where six or twelve anterior teeth were scored to measure tooth wear. To establish whether partial recording can be used for the measurement and reporting of tooth wear

Table 3. Localization of erosion in adults: a survey of different epidemiological studies listed in the order of the age of the examined samples

Author(s)	Year	Age (years)	Localization
Sognnaes et al. [36]	1972	–	Mandibular teeth (21%) with a higher frequency than the corresponding maxillary teeth (13%); with 28% Mandibular incisors showed the most lesions
Xhonga and Valdmanis [40]	1983	14–88	Minor erosions: premolars and anterior teeth Severe erosions: molars and premolars
Jaeggi et al. [41]	1999	19–25	Facial erosions: maxillary and mandibular canines and premolars Occlusal erosions: maxillary and mandibular first molars and premolars Palatal erosions: maxillary incisors and canines
Mathew et al. [44]	2002	18–28	Occlusal surface of mandibular first permanent molar most often affected (specific population study)
Ganss et al. [45]	1999	18–63	Facial erosions: anterior region of the maxillary jaw; canines and premolars of the mandibular jaw Occlusal erosions: most affected surfaces; evenly distributed (mandibular first molar) Palatal erosions: maxillary and mandibular anterior area (specific population study)
Lussi et al. [32]	1991	26–30 46–50	Facial erosions: maxillary and mandibular canines and premolars Occlusal erosions: maxillary and mandibular premolars and molars Palatal erosions: maxillary incisors and canines
Lussi et al. [42]	2000	32–36 52–56	Facial erosions: increase especially on premolar and molar surfaces Occlusal erosions: increase especially on canine, premolar and molar surfaces Palatal erosions: increase especially on maxillary central incisor surfaces

data in samples of adult populations, Steele and Walls [52] examined several different partial recording systems and compared them to the whole mouth coronal tooth wear data from a large random population sample of 1,211 dentate older adults in England (age 60 years or older). The 12 anterior teeth were the ones most often affected by moderate or severe wear, and when all 12 teeth were used as the index teeth, few wear cases were missed. They concluded that partial recording by screening six or twelve anterior teeth is appropriate for measuring tooth wear data in large population investigations.

A survey of the localization of erosion in adults is given in table 3. Prevalence and incidence data are summarized in table 4.

Table 4. Prevalence and incidence of erosion in adults (% of examined tooth surfaces): a survey of different epidemiological studies listed in the order of the age of the examined samples

Author(s)	Year	Sample		Examination	Erosion prevalence	Erosion incidence	Conclusion
		Age (years)	n				
Sognnaes et al. [36]	1972	–	10,827	Extracted teeth	18%[a]	–	Mandibular teeth (21%) with higher frequency of erosion than the corresponding maxillary teeth (13%)
Xhonga and Valdmanis [40]	1983	14–88	527	Clinical	25%[b]	–	Minor and severe erosions predominant
Johansson et al. [39]	1996	21	95	Clinical	28%[a]	–	Pronounced erosion (only maxillary anterior teeth were scored)
Jaeggi et al. [41]	1999	19–25	417	Clinical	F: 14.4%/0.5% O: 82.0%/30.7% P: 0.7%/0.0%	–	Prevalence data: enamel/dentinal erosions are listed F=facial, O=occlusal, P=palatal Occlusal erosions most frequent
Lussi et al. [32]	1991	26–30	194	Clinical	F: 11.9%/7.7% O: 35.6%/29.9% P: 3.6%/0.0%	–	Prevalence data: enamel/dentinal erosions are listed F=facial, O=occlusal, P=palatal
		46–50	197		F: 9.6%/13.2% O: 40.1%/42.6% P: 6.1%/2.0%		Increase of number and severity of erosive lesions with increasing age
Lussi and Schaffner [42]	2000	32–36 52–56	55	Clinical	O: 8% O: 26%	O: 5% O: 18%	O = occlusal erosions involving dentine Progression of erosion on facial and occlusal surfaces especially in the older age group
Smith and Robb [49]	1996	15–26 26–55 56–65 >65	1,007	Clinical	5.73% 3.37–4.62% 8.19% 8.84%	–	% of tooth surfaces with pathological level of tooth wear in relation to age (tooth wear study)

Table 4. (continued)

Author(s)	Year	Sample		Examination	Erosion prevalence	Erosion incidence	Conclusion
		Age (years)	n				
Schiffner et al. [43]	2002	35–44	655	Clinical	6.4%[b]/4.3%[b] (42.1%[b])	–	Prevalence data: facial enamel/dentinal erosions are listed
		65–74	1,027		4.1%[b]/3.8%[b] (46.3%[b])		(total of noncarious cervical lesions)

[a]% examined teeth; [b]% examined subjects.

Conclusions

As mentioned previously, it is difficult to make comparisons between studies, because of the different indices used and also because of the different teeth assessed in the sample. This is compounded by the multifactor nature of tooth wear. Tooth surface substance loss has different causes: erosion, attrition, abrasion and abfraction all contribute to the functional loss and aging of the teeth [53]. Prevalence data show that erosive tooth wear is a common condition. It can start as soon as the first dental surface reaches the oral cavity by exposure to extrinsic or intrinsic acid. Primary and permanent teeth are equally involved. If, in addition, mechanical stress loads the tooth surface, the progression of the defects increases further. Erosive tooth wear can be found on all tooth surfaces but is most common on occlusal and facial surfaces of all maxillary and mandibular teeth and on palatal surfaces of the maxillary anterior teeth.

Systematic (cross-sectional) prevalence data and incidence studies are scarce and, therefore, a conclusion about the occurrence, progression and distribution of erosive tooth wear cannot be made easily. There are some indications that the prevalence of erosive tooth wear shows an increase especially in younger age groups. The main explanation for this could be the change in nutritional habits and lifestyle. For the future, it is important to collect more data and obtain additional information about this condition. It would be of benefit if systematic investigations would be undertaken on all age groups, all social classes and the population of different geographic regions and cultures. Erosive tooth wear is a growing condition of the oral cavity and it is essential that adequate preventive measures are implemented on a risk group level.

References

1   Osatakul S, Sriplung H, Puetpaiboon A, Junjana CO, Chamnongpakdi S: Prevalence and natural course of gastroesophageal reflux symptoms: a 1-year cohort study in Thai infants. J Pediatr Gastroenterol Nutr 2002;34:63–67.
2   Järvinen VK, Rytömaa II, Heinonen OP: Risk factors in dental erosion. J Dent Res 1991;70: 942–947.
3   Linnet V, Seow WK: Dental erosion in children: a literature review. Pediatr Dent 2001;23:37–43.
4   Dahshan A, Patel H, Delaney J, Wuerth A, Thomas R, Tolia V: Gastroesophageal reflux disease and dental erosion in children. J Pediatr 2002;140:474–478.
5   O'Sullivan EA, Curzon ME, Roberts GJ, Milla PJ, Stringer MD: Gastroesophageal reflux in children and its relationship to erosion of primary and permanent teeth. Eur J Oral Sci 1998;106:765–769.
6   Lussi A, Jaeggi T, Zero D: The role of diet in the aetiology of dental erosion. Caries Res 2004;38: 34–44.
7   Dugmore CR, Rock WP: A multifactorial analysis of factors associated with dental erosion. Br Dent J 2004;196:283–286.
8   Hunter ML, West NX, Hughes JA, Newcombe RG, Addy M: Erosion of deciduous and permanent dental hard tissue in the oral environment. J Dent 2000;28:257–263.

9 Amaechi BT, Higham SM, Edgar WM: Factors influencing the development of dental erosion in vitro: enamel type, temperature and exposure time. J Oral Rehabil 1999;26:624–630.

10 Hunter ML, West NX, Hughes JA, Newcombe RG, Addy M: Relative susceptibility of deciduous and permanent dental hard tissues to erosion by a low pH fruit drink in vitro. J Dent 2000;28: 265–270.

11 Lussi A, Kohler N, Zero D, Schaffner M, Megert B: A comparison of the erosive potential of different beverages in primary and permanent teeth using an in vitro model. Eur J Oral Sci 2000;108: 110–114.

12 Lussi A, Schaffner M, Jaeggi T, Grüninger A: Erosionen: Befund – Diagnose – Risikofaktoren – Prävention – Therapie. Schweiz Monatsschr Zahnmed 2005;115:917–935.

13 Attin T, Koidl U, Buchalla W, Schaller HG, Kielbassa AM, Hellwig E: Correlation of microhardness and wear in differently eroded bovine dental enamel. Arch Oral Biol 1997;42:243–250.

14 Al-Malik MI, Holt RD, Bedi R: Erosion, caries and rampant caries in preschool children in Jeddah, Saudi Arabia. Community Dent Oral Epidemiol 2002;30:16–23.

15 Luo Y, Zeng XJ, Du MQ, Bedi R: The prevalence of dental erosion in preschool children in China. J Dent 2005;33:115–121.

16 Harding MA, Whelton H, O'Mullane DM, Cronin M: Dental erosion in 5-year-old Irish school children and associated factors: a pilot study. Community Dent Health 2003;20:165–170.

17 Millward A, Shaw L, Smith A: Dental erosion in four-year-old children from differing socioeconomic backgrounds. ASDC J Dent Child 1994;61:263–266.

18 Jaeggi T, Lussi A: Erosionen bei Kindern im frühen Schulalter. Schweiz Monatsschr Zahnmed 2004;114:876–881.

19 Ganss C, Klimek J, Giese K: Dental erosion in children and adolescents: a cross-sectional and longitudinal investigation using study models. Community Dent Oral Epidemiol 2001;29:264–271.

20 Truin GJ, Van Rijkom HM, Mulder J, Van't Hof MA: Caries Trends 1996–2002 among 6- and 12-year-old children and erosive wear prevalence among 12-year-old children in The Hague. Caries Res 2005;39:2–8.

21 Dugmore CR, Rock WP: The prevalence of tooth erosion in 12-year-old children. Br Dent J 2004;196:279–282.

22 Dugmore CR, Rock WP: The progression of tooth erosion in a cohort of adolescents of mixed ethnicity. Int J Paediatr Dent 2003;13:295–303.

23 Deery C, Wagner ML, Longbottom C, Simon R, Nugent ZJ: The prevalence of dental erosion in a United States and a United Kingdom sample of adolescents. Pediatr Dent 2000;22:505–510.

24 Chadwick RG, Mitchell HL, Manton SL, Ward S, Ogston S, Brown R: Maxillary incisor palatal erosion: no correlation with dietary variables? J Clin Pediatr Dent 2005;29:157–164.

25 Williams D, Croucher R, Marcenes W, O'Farrell M: The prevalence of dental erosion in the maxillary incisors of 14-year-old schoolchildren living in Tower Hamlets and Hackney, London, UK. Int Dent J 1999;49:211–216.

26 Bardsley PF, Taylor S, Milosevic A: Epidemiological studies of tooth wear and dental erosion in 14-year-old children in North West England. I. The relationship with water fluoridation and social deprivation. Br Dent J 2004;197:413–416.

27 Caglar E, Kargul B, Tanboga I, Lussi A: Dental erosion among children in an Istanbul public school. J Dent Child 2005;72:5–9.

28 Nunn JH, Rugg-Gunn A, Gordon PH, Stephenson G: A longitudinal study of dental erosion in adolescent girls. Caries Res 2001;35:296 (ORCA abstr. 97).

29 Milosevic A, Young PJ, Lennon MA: The prevalence of tooth wear in 14-year-old school children in Liverpool. Community Dent Health 1994;11:83–86.

30 Al-Dlaigan YH, Shaw L, Smith A: Dental erosion in a group of British 14-year-old, school children. I. Prevalence and influence of differing socioeconomic backgrounds. Br Dent J 2001;190:145–149.

31 Arnadottir IB, Saemundsson SR, Holbrook WP: Dental erosion in Icelandic teenagers in relation to dietary and lifestyle factors. Acta Odontol Scand 2003;61:25–28.

32 Lussi A, Schaffner M, Hotz P, Suter P: Dental erosion in a population of Swiss adults. Community Dent Oral Epidemiol 1991;19:286–290.

33 Van Rijkom HM, Truin GJ, Frencken JEFM, König KG, Van't Hof MA, Bronkhorst EM, Roeters FJM: Prevalence, distribution and background variables of smooth-bordered tooth wear in teenagers in The Hague, The Netherlands. Caries Res 2002;36:147–154.

34 Larsen MJ, Poulsen S, Hansen I: Erosion of the teeth: prevalence and distribution in a group of Danish school children. Eur J Paediatr Dent 2005;6:44–47.

35 Nunn JH, Gordon PH, Morris AJ, Pine CM, Walker A: Dental erosion – changing prevalence? A review of British national childrens' surveys. Int J Paediatr Dent 2003;13:98–105.

36 Sognnaes RF, Wolcott RB, Xhonga FA: Dental erosion. I. Erosion-like patterns occurring in association with other dental conditions. J Am Dent Assoc 1972;84:571–576.

37 Khan F, Young WG, Law V, Priest J, Daley TJ: Cupped lesions of early onset dental erosion in young southeast Queensland adults. Aust Dent J 2001;46:100–107.

38 Xhonga FA, Wolcott RB, Sognnaes RF: Dental erosion. II. Clinical measurements of dental erosion progress. J Am Dent Assoc 1972;84:577–582.

39 Johansson AK, Johansson A, Birkhed D, Omar R, Baghdadi S, Carlsson GE: Dental erosion, soft-drink intake, and oral health in young Saudi men, and the development of a system for assessing erosive anterior tooth wear. Acta Odontol Scand 1996;54:369–378.

40 Xhonga FA, Valdmanis S: Geographic comparisons of the incidence of dental erosion: a two centre study. J Oral Rehabil 1983;10:269–277.

41 Jaeggi T, Schaffner M, Bürgin W, Lussi A: Erosionen und keilförmige Defekte bei Rekruten der Schweizer Armee. Schweiz Monatsschr Zahnmed 1999;109:1171–1182.

42 Lussi A, Schaffner M: Progression of and risk factors for dental erosion and wedge-shaped defects over a 6-year period. Caries Res 2000;34:182–187.

43 Schiffner U, Micheelis W, Reich E: Erosionen und keilförmige Zahnhalsdefekte bei deutschen Erwachsenen und Senioren. Dtsch Zahnärztl Z 2002;57:102–106.

44 Mathew T, Casamassimo PS, Hayes JR: Relationship between sports drinks and dental erosion in 304 university athletes in Columbus, Ohio, USA. Caries Res 2002;36:281–287.

45 Ganss C, Schlechtriemen M, Klimek J: Dental erosions in subjects living on a raw food diet. Caries Res 1999;33:74–80.

46 Tuominen ML, Tuominen RJ, Fubusa F, Mgalula N: Tooth surface loss and exposure to organic and inorganic acid fumes in workplace air. Community Dent Oral Epidemiol 1991;19:217–220.

47 Smith BGN, Knight JK: An index for measuring the wear of teeth. Br Dent J 1984;156:435–438.

48 Donachie MA, Walls AW: The tooth wear index: a flawed epidemiological tool in an ageing population group. Community Dent Oral Epidemiol 1996;24:152–158.

49 Smith BG, Robb ND: The prevalence of tooth wear in 1,007 dental patients. J Oral Rehabil 1996;23:232–239.

50 Ekfeld A: Incisal and occlusal tooth wear and wear of some prosthodontic materials: an epidemiological and clinical study. Swed Dent J Suppl 1989;65:1–62.

51 Donachie MA, Walls AWG: Assessment of tooth wear in an ageing population. J Dent 1995;23:157–164.

52 Steele JG, Walls AWG: Using partial recording to assess tooth wear in older adults. Community Dent Oral Epidemiol 2000;28:18–25.

53 Nunn JH: Prevalence of dental erosion and the implications for oral health. Eur J Oral Sci 1996;104:156–161.

Dr. Thomas Jaeggi
Department of Preventive, Restorative and Pediatric Dentistry
School of Dental Medicine
University of Bern
Freiburgstrasse 7
CH–3010 Bern (Switzerland)

Lussi A (ed): Dental Erosion.
Monogr Oral Sci. Basel, Karger, 2006, vol 20, pp 66–76

· ·

Understanding the Chemistry of Dental Erosion

J.D.B. Featherstone[a], Adrian Lussi[b]

[a]Department of Preventive and Restorative Dental Sciences, University of California at San Francisco, San Francisco, Calif., USA; [b]Department of Preventive, Restorative and Paediatric Dentistry, School of Dental Medicine, University of Bern, Bern, Switzerland

Abstract

The mineral in our teeth is composed of a calcium-deficient carbonated hydroxyapatite $(Ca_{10-x} Na_x (PO_4)_{6-y} (CO_3)_z (OH)_{2-u} F_u)$. These substitutions in the mineral crystal lattice, especially carbonate, renders tooth mineral more acid soluble than hydroxyapatite. During erosion by acid and/or chelators, these agents interact with the surface of the mineral crystals, but only after they diffuse through the plaque, the pellicle, and the protein/lipid coating of the individual crystals themselves. The effect of direct attack by the hydrogen ion is to combine with the carbonate and/or phosphate releasing all of the ions from that region of the crystal surface leading to direct surface etching. Acids such as citric acid have a more complex interaction. In water they exist as a mixture of hydrogen ions, acid anions (e.g. citrate) and undissociated acid molecules, with the amounts of each determined by the acid dissociation constant (pK_a) and the pH of the solution. Above the effect of the hydrogen ion, the citrate ion can complex with calcium also removing it from the crystal surface and/or from saliva. Values of the strength of acid (pK_a) and for the anion–calcium interaction and the mechanisms of interaction with the tooth mineral on the surface and underneath are described in detail.

Our objective is to provide a model for the chemical understanding of dental erosion. With a true understanding of the mechanisms involved, it is possible to readily interpret observations both in research and in the clinic, and most importantly as the basis for preventive interventions and therapy for patients. The chemistry behind erosion is the key to embracing the information in this publication and putting it into practice in the real world.

First, we must review the chemical nature of enamel and dentine since this is the substrate upon which erosive agents have their effect.

Table 1. Approximate composition of enamel and dentine as volume percent of total tissue [1, 2]

Component	Enamel percent by volume	Dentine percent by volume
Carbonated hydroxyapatide	85	47
Water	12	20
Protein and lipid	3	33

Enamel and Dentine Composition

Dental enamel and dentine consist of mineral, protein, lipid and water [1–3]. The two tissues are very different in their structure, while at the same time having similar components. Each is comprised of millions of tiny crystals laid down in a water/organic matrix. Dental enamel is approximately 96% by weight mineral, but more importantly if the components are calculated by percent volume instead, it is obvious that the organic and water components play an important role even in enamel compared with dentine. Molecules diffuse through the water/protein/lipid matrix that surrounds the mineral crystals. Table 1 presents approximate composition for enamel and dentine as volume percent of each of the components, as reviewed by Curzon and Featherstone [2].

The mineral in our teeth and bones is composed of a highly substituted hydroxyapatite (HAP), better described as a calcium-deficient carbonated HAP [4]. A simplified formula that helps to illustrate this is $Ca_{10-x} Na_x (PO_4)_{6-y} (CO_3)_z (OH)_{2-u} F_u$ in contrast to HAP which has the perfect formula $Ca_{10} (PO_4)_6 (OH)_2$. Tooth mineral is calcium deficient, as indicated by the $10-x$ after the Ca in the formula. Some calcium ions are replaced by other metal ions, such as sodium, magnesium and potassium totaling approximately 1%, with sodium (Na) being the most abundant. Some of the OH^- ions can be replaced by F^-. However, the major substitution is carbonate (CO_3) that replaces some of the phosphate (PO_4) but not on a one/one (stoichiometric) basis, hence the phosphate is designated as $6-y$ and the carbonate as z. These substitutions in the mineral crystal lattice, especially carbonate, disturb the structure [4, 5]. Because of these substitutions the mineral in enamel and dentine is much more acid soluble than HAP (see fig. 2), which in turn is much more soluble than fluorapatite (FAP) which has the formula $Ca_{10} (PO_4)_6 F_2$ [1, 4, 6]. Dentine and enamel have similar mineral compositions, although the carbonate content is much higher in dentine. The carbonate content of enamel is approximately 3% while in dentine it is 5–6%, making dentine mineral even more acid soluble. Further, the crystals in dentine are much smaller than those in enamel, therefore the surface area per gram dentine is much higher giving more surface available for acid attack.

The proteins in enamel (table 1) are primarily present as a very thin covering on the individual crystals and comprise approximately half of the organic material. The other half of the organic material in the enamel is lipid [7]. The water content of enamel is sufficient for diffusion of acids and other components into the tooth and of mineral (calcium and phosphate) out of the tooth during the erosion process [8]. In contrast, dentine has different proteins and a large component of the tissue is collagen type I with about 10% of the protein comprised of a range of noncollagenous proteins, such as phosphoproteins, proteoglycans and Gla proteins [9]. There is also about 1% by weight of lipid in dentine [7]. As can be seen from table 1, the water content of dentine is substantial.

During erosion by acid and/or chelators these agents interact with the surface of the mineral crystals but only after they diffuse through the plaque (if there is plaque present), through the pellicle (see below), and through the protein/lipid coating on the individual crystals themselves.

Acids and Chelating Agents

Chemical erosion of the teeth occurs either by the hydrogen ion derived from strong/weak acids, or by anions which can bind or complex calcium. The latter are known as chelating agents. It is rare that a simple inorganic acid, such as hydrochloric acid, is present in the mouth. Mostly, we are concerned with so-called weak acids, such as citric and acetic acid.

The hydrogen ions, H^+, are derived from acids as they dissociate in water. For example, citric acid (fig. 1) has the possibility of producing three hydrogen ions from each molecule. The H^+ ion itself can attack the tooth mineral crystals and directly dissolve by combining with either the carbonate ion or the phosphate ion, as shown in equation (1).

$$Ca_{10-x} Na_x (PO_4)_{6-y} (CO_3)_z (OH)_{2-u} F_u + 3H^+ \rightarrow$$
$$(10-x)Ca^{2+} + xNa^+ + (6-y)(HPO_4^{2-}) + z(HCO_3^-) + H_2O + uF^- \qquad (1)$$

The effect of direct attack by the hydrogen ion is to combine with the carbonate and/or phosphate releasing all of the ions from that region of the crystal surface leading to direct surface etching. For example, hydrochloric acid, which dissociates completely in water to hydrogen ions and chloride ions, rapidly and directly dissolves and removes the mineral surface. The chloride ion plays no role in the mineral dissolution process.

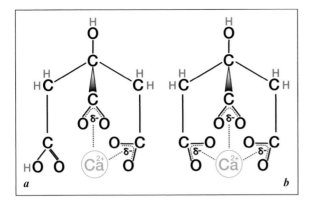

Fig. 1. Schematic representation of citrate ion chelating a calcium ion. The diagram represent the situation where two of the COOH groups have lost the hydrogen and are negatively charged, thereby attracting the positively charged calcium ion (***a***). In the basic pH range even three COOH groups may have lost the hydrogen (***b***).

Table 2. Acid dissociation constants ($pK_a = -\log K_a$, where K_a is the acid dissociation constant) and calcium association constants (where log K* is the stability constant with calcium ion) for selected acids and chelating agents (thermodynamic values for 25°C except where indicated) [in part from 18]

Acid	pK_{a1}	pK_{a2}	pK_{a3}	log $K_{Ca}(1)$	log $K_{Ca}(2)$	log $K_{Ca}(3)$
Acetic	4.76			1.18		
Lactic	3.86			1.45		
Citric	3.13	4.76	6.40	1.10	3.09	4.68
Phosphoric	2.15	7.20	12.35	1.40	2.74	6.46
Tartaric	3.04	4.37		0.92**	2.80	
Carbonic	6.35	10.33		1.00	3.15	
Oxalic	1.25	4.27		1.84	3.00***	
EDTA				10.7		

*Higher numbers indicate stronger binding.
**Temperature not stated, ionic strength 0.2.
***18°C, zero ionic strength.

Acids such as citric acid (fig. 1) have a more complex interaction. In water they exist as a mixture of hydrogen ions, acid anions (e.g. citrate) and undissociated acid molecules, with the amounts of each determined by the acid dissociation constant and the pH of the solution. The hydrogen ion behaves exactly as described above and directly attacks the crystal surface. Over and above the effect of the hydrogen ion the citrate anion may complex with calcium also removing it from the crystal surface. Each acid anion has a different strength of calcium complexation dependent on the structure of the molecule and how easily it can attract the calcium ion (fig. 1). Consequently, acids such as citric have double actions and are very damaging to the tooth surface.

The strength of acids are given by their acid dissociation constant (K_a) values. The most useful way of describing the strength of acids is the pK_a value (table 2) which is the negative logarithm of the K_a value. When the pH value (acidity) of a solution equals the pK_a of a weak acid the acid exists as 50% anion and 50% undissociated acid molecule, providing hydrogen ions to the solution. In the case of erosion as the hydrogen ions interact with the apatite mineral the acid equilibrium shifts providing more hydrogen ions to continue the erosion. Equation (2) illustrates the equilibrium for such acids using acetic acid as an example:

$$CH_3COOH \leftrightarrow CH_3COO^- + H^+ \tag{2}$$

The stability constant (K) for the anion–calcium interaction is a measure of the strength of this interaction. Increasing values of $\log K$ (table 2) indicate a stronger bond. Citric acid is much more damaging to the mineral than acetic acid from the perspective of calcium binding. The stronger the bond, the more likely the anion is to pull calcium from the apatite mineral surface and into solution, i.e. to erode the crystal surface. Dental erosion is a combination of the mineral being dissolved by attack from the hydrogen ion and mineral dissolving by calcium being complexed by anions, especially those with strong chelating action such as citric acid and EDTA (table 2). EDTA is a well known chelating agent that is used to demineralize bone and teeth samples for histological evaluation. EDTA can demineralize at neutral pH because of the strength of the binding with calcium ions (table 2).

For weak acids, such as acetic acid, as the hydrogen ions are used up in their interaction with the apatite the equilibrium shifts to the right (eq. (2)) continually providing hydrogen ions until all the acid is used up. This describes chemically how acetic acid erosion in the form of vinegar works to dissolve the teeth as reported by Lussi et al. [10] for salad dressing erosion. In the case of acetic acid, the calcium/acetate formation is very weak and plays little part in erosion. On the other hand, lactic acid binds stronger to calcium because of the added OH side group on the molecule. Lactic acid ($pK_a = 3.86$) is also stronger than acetic

Table 3. Acid composition of different beverages (g/l)

Beverage	pH	Phosphoric acid	Citric acid	D-isocitric acid	Malic acid	Miscellaneous acids
Pineapple juice	3.4–3.5		5.9		1.3	Salicylic: 0.16
Apple juice, fresh	3.0–3.4		0.05–2	0.01	7.4	Lactic: 0.17 Formic: 0.02
Cola beverage	2.2–2.6	3.3	9			Carbonic: 4–6
Grapefruit juice, fresh	3.2–3.4		13.9	194	0.44	
Orange juice, fresh	3.4–3.7		7.6–11.9	0.1	1.1–2.9	
Red wine	3.4–3.7				0.3–5.1	Lactic: 2.4 Tartaric: 1.5
White wine	3.4–3.7		0.14		3.5	Lactic: 1.7 Tartaric: 0.3

acid ($pK_a = 4.76$) therefore providing hydrogen ions more readily, producing a lower pH in solution and behaving similarly to equation (2) for acetic acid. However, lactate also binds calcium. Interestingly, because of this, lactic acid can erode dental enamel even at pH 6–7, where there is almost no hydrogen ion present and the etching is due to binding of calcium with the lactate ion [11].

Citric acid is even more complicated. It has three pK_a values, one for each of the hydrogen ions reversibly bound to the citrate ion (table 2), as illustrated in figure 1 and equation (3):

$$HOOCCH_2COH(COOH)CH_2COOH \leftrightarrow HOOCCH_2COH(COOH)CH_2COO^-$$
$$\leftrightarrow {}^-OOCCH_2COH(COOH)CH_2COO^- \leftrightarrow {}^-OOCCH_2COH(COO^-)CH_2COO^- \quad (3)$$

The citrate ion can exist in each of the forms shown in equation (3), and when two or even all of the three H's have been removed from the molecule it forms a complex with calcium by a three-dimensional electrostatic interaction from each of the COO^- groups to the calcium ion (fig. 1; eq. (3)), thereby acting as a so-called chelator. This form will only occur in basic pH values. This means that citric acid at lower pH, such as 2, provides hydrogen ions to directly attack the mineral surface and at higher pH, such as 7, the citrate ion draws the calcium out of the crystal surface. At intermediate pH values both mechanisms are in place. In the case of fruits and fruit juices (table 3) which are high in citric acid many reports of erosion are in the literature (see chapter 7.1.1 by Lussi et al., this vol, pp 77–87).

Phosphoric acid has three pK_a values and further binds to calcium in solution (table 2). Phosphoric acid provides hydrogen ions at low pH, such as 2, and binds calcium at higher pH, such as 7. In between, both mechanisms are in effect, just as with citric acid. Citrate, however, forms a complex with calcium because of the relative sizes and three-dimensional shapes of the molecules.

Acid Interactions with the Mineral

Figure 2 shows the solubility lines (so-called isotherms) for enamel mineral, HAP and FAP versus the pH, taking into consideration the concentrations of calcium and phosphate in the solution. The vertical axis is the negative logarithm of the combined total concentrations of calcium and phosphate, in any solution, which could be in saliva, in plaque fluid, in the aqueous film on the surface of the tooth, or inside the enamel or dentine. The enamel line is above the HAP line, which in turn is above the FAP line, indicating orders of magnitude differences in solubility between each of these. Dentine (not shown for clarity) is even higher in solubility than enamel. Calcium and phosphate combinations above any line are so-called 'supersaturated' with respect to that mineral and cannot dissolve. Below the line they are 'undersaturated' and dissolves. This means that if we start at a point on the enamel surface step 1 (fig. 2) indicates changing to a lower the pH, and because the solution is undersaturated with respect to enamel mineral must dissolve until the concentration increases back to the enamel solubility line (step 2). As the pH is raised by buffering from saliva (step 3; fig. 2) the solution becomes supersaturated and new mineral can form on the crystal surface (step 4; fig. 2). If fluoride is present FAP can form, which has a much lower solubility than the original enamel as described in more detail below. The additional importance of this diagram is that if the concentrations of calcium and/or phosphate are increased at any pH it is possible to be above the solubility line and to stop dissolution of the crystals. With respect to erosion it is therefore possible to add calcium and or phosphate to food and beverages, such as orange juice or black currant juice, and to protect against the erosion caused by the citric acid content. Further, the added calcium can complex with the citrate also inhibiting the chelation effect described above.

It is possible after an erosion challenge to remineralize a softened subsurface provided it has not been directly etched away. Saliva buffers the acid returning the pH to neutral, as illustrated by step 3 in figure 2. In this case calcium and phosphate from saliva or other sources can now cause remineralization, and in the presence of sufficient fluoride a new mineral surface forms which is much less soluble in acid (step 4; fig. 2). However if a severe erosion challenge follows it can still overcome the protection and directly erode the surface, especially if a chelator, such as citric acid is present.

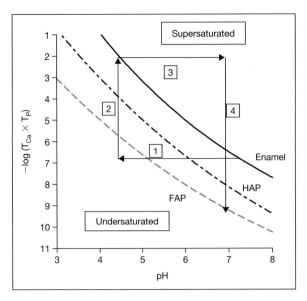

Fig. 2. Solubility lines for enamel, HAP and FAP. T_{Ca} and T_P are the total concentrations of calcium and phosphate in solution, respectively. The numbered steps represent stages in mineral loss by acid attack, namely lowering the pH from say 7.3 to 4.5 at the enamel surface as the acid beverage attacks the tooth surface (step 1), and dissolving calcium and phosphate (step 2). Step 3 is when saliva flows over the affected area and the pH rises to say 7.0. If fluoride is present, together with saliva the softened surface is repaired (step 4), at least partially, forming a mineral surface closer to FAP which then requires a larger pH drop to be dissolved. If fluoride is not present then the step 4 line stops at the enamel line, and the cycle simply repeats itself and the tooth mineral continues to dissolve.

Pellicle and Diffusion Barriers

As soon as the tooth erupts into the mouth a salivary pellicle begins to form on the surface. The pellicle is derived from specific salivary proteins and lipids that bind to the surface of the tooth [12, 13]. The salivary proteins such as statherin, proline rich proteins, some histatins, and phospholipids comprise the initial pellicle [14]. The pellicle is continually regenerated throughout the life of the tooth in the mouth. The net effect with respect to erosion is that the pellicle forms a diffusion barrier, similar to a lipid/protein membrane, and protects the very outer surface against direct acid attack. The plaque bacteria build upon the pellicle, forming a further diffusion barrier, wherever plaque is present (see chapter 7.1.2 by Hara et al., this vol, pp 88–99). On smooth accessible surfaces there is often little or no plaque leaving only the pellicle as the first barrier to

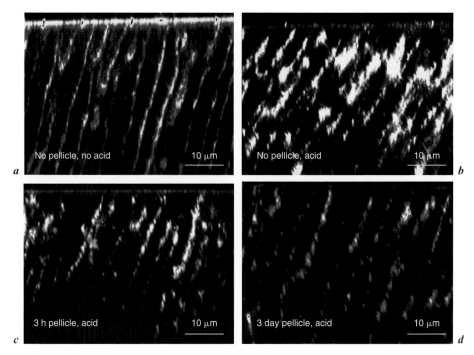

Fig. 3. a Optical section perpendicular to the surface of sound enamel made with the confocal laser scanning microscope. Light-yellowish area represent interprismatic enamel, red areas represent prismatic area. From Duschner et al. [15], with permission. **b** After 15 min immersion in a Cola-like beverage the enamel was removed and dissolved underneath the surface (in the subsurface region). Further, hardness measurement showed distinct softening of the surface. **c** Image of enamel after a pellicle was formed for 3 h and 15 min immersion in a Cola-like beverage. The band-like structure of enamel can be identified indicating partial protection against subsurface dissolution. Hardness measurement showed still softening of the surface. **d** Image of enamel after a pellicle was formed for 3 days. The band-like structure of enamel can be clearly identified with only small differences to the control. Hardness measurement showed no significant softening of the surface.

acid erosion. At the gingival margin there is almost always plaque and crevicular fluid access thereby protecting a narrow band from erosion.

To investigate these aspects experiments were done with and without pellicle present [15]. Figure 3 illustrates, using confocal microscopy, the partial protective effect of pellicle against erosion. In these experiments enamel samples, with or without pellicle, were immersed for 15 min in a Cola type beverage, pH 2.6, which included phosphoric acid. The control panel shows no erosion. Without pellicle, removal and surface softening of enamel was observed together with dissolution underneath the surface (in the subsurface region) (fig. 3b).

When pellicle was formed over 3 h, the surface was still softened, but there was partial protection against subsurface dissolution (fig. 3c). The samples with 3-day pellicle markedly reduced surface softening and essentially eliminated subsurface attack. These observations can be interpreted using the information set out above for phosphoric acid. At pH 2.6 the hydrogen ion concentration is such that direct etching occurs by the hydrogen ion in the absence of pellicle since there is nothing to protect the surface. In the case of the 3-h pellicle it is not sufficient to protect the outer surface but it does form a partial diffusion barrier to the subsurface. In this case, the phosphoric acid molecule is able to diffuse in its undissociated state into the subsurface region [8, 16], dissociating as it goes providing hydrogen ions and phosphate ions to attack the mineral. In the case of the 3-day mature pellicle there was considerable surface protection as expected form earlier studies that showed protection increased after 18 h and took 7 days to be essentially complete [17]. Importantly, the 3-day pellicle markedly reduced the ability of even the phosphoric acid molecule to diffuse into the subsurface regions.

The conclusions from the pellicle experiments described above are clinically significant because they illustrate how important the type of acid is and whether there is a pellicle present from the saliva. Further, if the dental erosion lesion has a subsurface softening component rather than direct etching alone there is a chance for repair and reversal, since the saliva can provide calcium and phosphate to remineralize these regions, aided by fluoride. Salivary pellicle can partially protect against erosion challenges providing they are not too severe and/or frequent. Saliva also clears the erosion-inducing acids from the surface, but again the eventual outcome depends on the balance between the frequency and severity of the erosion challenge versus the protective effects of saliva.

References

1   Featherstone JDB: The science and practice of caries prevention. J Am Dent Assoc 2000;131: 887–899.
2   Curzon MEJ, Featherstone JDB: Chemical composition of enamel; in Lazzari EP (ed): Handbook of Experimental Aspects of Oral Biochemistry. Boca Raton, CRC Press, 1983, pp 123–135.
3   Linde A: Dentine: structure, chemistry and formation; in Thylstrup A, Leach SA, Qvist V (eds): Dentine and Dentine Reactions in the Oral Cavity. Oxford, IRL Press, 1983, pp 17–26.
4   LeGeros RZ: Calcium phosphates in enamel, dentine and bone; in Myers HM (ed): Calcium Phosphates in Oral Biology and Medicine. Basel, Karger, 1991, vol 15, pp 108–129.
5   Featherstone JDB, Mayer I, Driessens FCM, Verbeeck RMH, Heijligers HJM: Synthetic apatites containing Na, Mg, and CO₃ and their comparison with tooth enamel mineral. Calcif Tissue Int 1983;35:169–171.
6   Featherstone JDB, Shields CP, Khademazad B, Oldershaw MD: Acid reactivity of carbonated-apatites with strontium and fluoride substitutions. J Dent Res 1983;62:1049–1053.
7   Odutuga AA, Prout RES: Lipid analysis of human enamel and dentine. Archs Oral Biol 1974;19: 729–731.

8 Featherstone JDB: Diffusion phenomena and enamel caries development; in Guggenheim (ed): International Congress in Honour of Professor Dr. H.R. Mühlemann, Zürich, 1983, pp 259–268.

9 Linde A: Dentine: structure, chemistry, and formation; in Thylstrup A, Qvist V (ed): Dentine and Dentine Reactions in the Oral Cavity. Oxford, IRL Press, 1987, pp 17–26.

10 Lussi A, Jaeggi T, Schaerer S: The influence of different factors on in vitro enamel erosion. Caries Res 1993;27:387–393.

11 Featherstone JDB, Duncan JF, Cutress TW: A mechanism for dental caries based on chemical processes and diffusion phenomena during in vitro caries simulation on human tooth enamel. Arch Oral Biol 1979;24:101–112.

12 Mandel ID: The role of saliva in maintaining oral homeostasis. J Am Dent Assoc 1989;119:298–304.

13 Moreno EC, Kresak M, Hay DI: Adsorption of molecules of biological interest onto hydroxyapatite. Calcif Tissue Int 1984;36:48–59.

14 Lamkin MS, Oppenheim FG: Structural features of salivary function. Crit Rev Oral Biol Med 1993;4:251–259.

15 Duschner H, Götz H, Walker R, Lussi A: Erosion of dental enamel visualized by confocal laser scanning microscopy; in Addy M, Embery G, Edgar WM, Orchardson R (eds): Tooth Wear and Sensitivity. London, Martin Dunitz, 2000, pp 67–73.

16 Featherstone JDB, Rodgers BE: The effect of acetic, lactic and other organic acids on the formation of artificial carious lesions. Caries Res 1981;15:377–385.

17 Featherstone JDB, Behrman JM, Bell JE: Effect of whole saliva components on enamel demineralization in vitro. Crit Rev Oral Biol Med 1993;4:357–362.

18 Smith RM, Martell AE: Critical stability constants; in Smith RM, Martell AE. New York, London: Plenum Press, 1974.

Prof. Dr. J.D.B. Featherstone
Department of Preventive and Restorative Dental Sciences
University of California at San Francisco
Room 0603, Box 0758
707 Parnassus Avenue
San Francisco, CA 94143 (USA)

Lussi A (ed): Dental Erosion.
Monogr Oral Sci. Basel, Karger, 2006, vol 20, pp 77–87

....

Chemical Factors

Adrian Lussi, Thomas Jaeggi

Department of Preventive, Restorative and Pediatric Dentistry,
School of Dental Medicine, University of Bern, Bern, Switzerland

Abstract

pH value, calcium, and phosphate and to a lesser extent fluoride content of a drink or
foodstuff are important factors explaining erosive attack. They determine the degree of saturation with respect to tooth minerals, which is the driving force for dissolution. Solutions
oversaturated with respect to dental hard tissue will not dissolve it. Addition of calcium (and
phosphate) salts to erosive drinks showed protection of surface softening. Today, several Ca-
enriched soft drinks are on the market or products with naturally high content in Ca and P are
available (such as yoghurt), which do not soften the dental hard tissue. The greater the buffering capacity of the drink or food, the longer it will take for the saliva to neutralize the acid.
The buffer capacity of a solution has a distinct effect on the erosive attack when the solution
remains adjacent to the tooth surface and is not replaced by saliva. A higher buffer capacity
of a drink or foodstuff will enhance the processes of dissolution because more ions from the
tooth mineral are needed to render the acid inactive for further demineralization. Further, the
amount of drink in the mouth in relation to the amount of saliva present will modify the
process of dissolution. There is no clear-cut critical pH for erosion as there is for caries. Even
at a low pH, it is possible that other factors are strong enough to prevent erosion.

Chemical Factors

This chapter is aimed at revealing the interplay between the erosive potential
of food and beverages and their chemical properties. The term 'chemical factors'
is used to describe parameters inherent to erosive beverages, food or other products (table 1). Several in vitro and in situ studies on humans as well as on animals
have evaluated the erosive potential of different food and beverages [1–14]. They
all show that the erosive potential of an acidic drink is not exclusively dependent
on its pH value, but is also strongly influenced by its mineral content, its titratable
acidity ('the buffering capacity') and by the calcium-chelation properties of the

Table 1. Chemical factors influencing the erosive potential with respect to food and beverages

---

- pH and buffering capacity of the product
- Type of acid (pK$_a$ values)
- Adhesion of the product to the dental surface
- Chelating properties of the product
- Calcium concentration
- Phosphate concentration
- Fluoride concentration

---

food and beverages (see chapter 6 by Featherstone et al., this vol, pp 66–76). The pH value, calcium, phosphate and fluoride content of a drink or foodstuff determine the degree of saturation with respect to the tooth mineral, which is the driving force for dissolution. Solutions oversaturated with respect to dental hard tissue will not dissolve it. A low degree of undersaturation with respect to enamel or dentine leads to a very initial surface demineralization which is followed by a local rise in pH and increased mineral content in the liquid surface layer adjacent to the tooth surface. This layer will then become saturated with respect to enamel (or dentine) and will not demineralize further. Consequently, no softening can be measured with most of the methods used nowadays. An increase in agitation (e.g. when a patient is swishing his/her drink in the mouth) will enhance the dissolution process because the solution on the surface layer adjacent to tooth mineral will be readily renewed. When an excess of an erosive agent is present the pH is probably the most decisive factor whereas the buffering capacity is more important at the liquid surface layer adjacent to the tooth surface and/or when there is only a small amount of acid present around the tooth surface. Further, the amount of drink in the mouth in relation to the amount of saliva present will modify the dissolution process.

The chelating properties of citric acid (for example) can enhance the erosive process in vivo by interacting with saliva as well as directly soften and dissolving tooth mineral. Up to 32% of the calcium in saliva can be complexed by citrate at concentrations common in fruit juices, thus reducing the super saturation of saliva and increasing the driving force for dissolution with respect to tooth minerals [15]. In addition, calcium-chelating agents may directly dissolve tooth mineral. The greater the buffering capacity of the drink, the longer it will take for saliva to neutralize the acid. Some beverages appear to be less erosive than others within the same pH class. It may also be possible to reduce the erosive potential of beverages by modifying the amount and type of acid used in formulations, e.g., using maleic acid instead of citric acid [16]. In experiments conducted in vitro, citric acid caused more erosion than phosphoric acid at comparable acidity [17]. The erosive character of different pure acids at pH 2, 2.3 and 3 during incubation of bovine enamel between 1 and 5 min was high for lactic acid and lower for maleic and hydrochloric acid compared to other tested acids (acetic, citric, oxalic, phosphoric and tartaric acid) [18]. Diluting drinks containing organic acids with high buffering capacity with water will hardly reduce the pH but will reduce the relative titratable acidity. But dilution will also reduce the concentrations of Ca and P (if present), which have a protective effect [9, 19, 20].

The calcium and phosphate contents of a foodstuff or beverage are important factors for the erosive potential as they influence the concentration gradient within the local environment of the tooth surface. Indeed, addition of calcium (and phosphate) salts to erosive drinks showed promising results. Larsen [21] suggested that erosion potential could be calculated based on the degree of saturation with respect to both hydroxyapatite and fluorapatite by determining the pH, calcium, phosphate and fluoride content of a beverage. Orange juice (pH 4) supplemented with calcium (42.9 mmol/l) and phosphate (31.2 mmol/l) did not erode enamel after immersion for 7 days [22]. Only a small change in the degree of saturation by adding Ca (and a small amount of phosphate), without changing the pH may reduce the erosive potential in vitro [23]. One percent citric acid solution (pH 2.2) supplemented with different concentrations of calcium, phosphate and/or fluoride reduced the erosive potential of the solution [24]. The same was true when soft drinks were modified with calcium, phosphate and/or fluoride. The most effective reduction of enamel dissolution was achieved by adding either 1.0 mmol/l calcium or a combination of 0.5 mmol/l calcium plus 0.5 mmol/l phosphate plus 0.031 mmol/l fluoride to the citric acid [25].

It has to be kept in mind that with the added mineral enamel dissolution could not always be completely prevented. But the progression can be retarded which has some implications for the patient and the clinician.

Today, several Ca-enriched orange juices are on the market which hardly soften the enamel surface (fig. 1). Addition of calcium to a low pH blackcurrant juice drink has been shown to reduce the erosive effect of the drink [26]. In a follow-up study, a blackcurrant drink with added calcium was compared to a conventional orange drink in situ. Servings of 250 ml of each drink were consumed four times per day during 20 working days. Measurements of enamel loss were made by profilometry on enamel samples for up to 20 days. The experimental carbonated blackcurrant drink supplemented with calcium caused significantly less enamel loss than the conventional carbonated orange drink at all time points measured [27].

Sports drinks are often erosive [13, 28–30] and when consumed during strenuous activity when the person is in a state of some dehydration, the possible destructive effects may be enhanced further. A calcium-enriched experimental

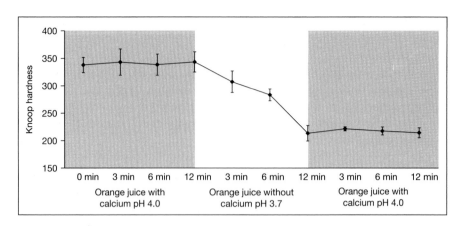

Fig. 1. Impact of a conventional and a Ca-enriched orange juice on softening of enamel.

Table 2. Content of some minimally erosive beverages (ready to drink) [in part from 30, 46]

Available beverage	pH	Added level of calcium (mg/l)
Ribena really light blackcurrant[a]	3.7–4.0	630
Ribena really light apple[a]	3.7–4.0	440
Ribena really light berry burst[a]	3.7–4.0	400
Ribena really light strawberry[a]	3.7–4.0	400
Ribena really light orange tropical[a]	3.7–4.0	200
Lucozade sport hydroactive citrus fruits (and summer) flavor[a]	3.7–4.0	370
Orange-flavored sports drinks[b]	3.8	320
Orange juice Michel[c]	3.8	160

[a]GlaxoSmithKline, Coleford, GB.
[b]Novartis Consumer Health, Basel, Switzerland.
[c]Rivella, Rothrist, Switzerland.

sports drink consumed during controlled sporting activities showed only minimal erosion compared with a commercially available sports drink [29]. A recently published study [31] showed a significant reduction of the erosive potential of a sports drink when phosphopeptide-stabilized amorphous calcium phosphate was added. As mentioned above, the pH increased and the titratable acid decreased with increasing phosphopeptide stabilized amorphous calcium phosphate concentrations. The same was true when Ca was added to another brand of sports drink (table 2) [30]. Yoghurt is another example of a food with a low pH (~4.0), yet it has hardly any erosive effect due to its high calcium and phosphate content, which makes it supersaturated with respect to apatite. A yoghurt or another milk-based food may have an erosive potential, when it has a low content of Ca and/or P and a low pH. It seems that the reduction in enamel dissolution caused by a minor increase in pH is likely to be small [32].

Larsen and Nyvad [22] and Larsen and Richards [33] reported that fluoride is unable to reduce dental erosion. Theoretically, fluoride has some protective effect in a drink with a pH higher than that indicated by the saturation curve of fluorapatite at given Ca and PO_4 concentrations. Lussi et al. [9, 20] and Mahoney et al. [34] found an inverse correlation of the erosive potential with fluoride content of different beverages. It is unlikely that fluoride at the concentration present in beverages alone has any great beneficial effect on erosion, because the challenge is high. However, it is possible that under conditions in which the other erosive factors are not excessive, fluoride in solution may exert some protective effect [34]. Due to health concerns, adding fluoride to drinks is not practical. After an initial demineralization, an intensive fluoridation is capable of inhibiting the erosive mineral loss in dentine completely. This is probably due to the buffering capacity of the proteins in the dentine matrix [35].

Table 3 gives an overview of the chemical properties of different beverages and foodstuffs. The pH, the titratable acid to pH 7.0, phosphorus and calcium concentration, fluoride content, and the degree of saturation with respect to hydroxyapatite as well as to fluorapatite are given. The methods used were as follows [9]: Caries-free human premolars with no cracks on the buccal sites were ground flat under water-cooling on a rotating polishing machine (Knuth-Rotor, Struers, Copenhagen, Denmark). The procedure was such that 200 μm of tooth substance in the center of the window was polished away. To quantify the softening of the enamel, measurement of surface microhardness (SMH), using a Knoop diamond under a load of 50 g, was performed before and after immersion for 3 or 20 min in the foodstuffs and beverages [9, 20]. A positive value denotes a hardening of the surface while a negative value represents softening. All substances were analyzed for phosphorus, calcium and fluoride using standard procedures. The pH and the amount of base added to raise the pH to 7.0 were measured using a pH electrode. To do so, 50 ml of each substance was titrated with NaOH and the amount of base added (mmol/l) was calculated.

The degrees of saturation (pK–pl) with respect to hydroxyapatite and fluorapatite were calculated using a computer program developed and later modified by Larsen [36]. This program assumes a solubility product for hydroxyapatite of $10^{-58.5}$ [37], for fluorapatite of $10^{-59.6}$, for calcium fluoride of $10^{-10.5}$ [38]. Orange juice, for example is undersaturated with respect to both hydroxyapatite and fluorapatite as expressed by pK–pl, and caused surface softening in the

Table 3. pH, titratable acid, inorganic phosphorus, calcium and fluoride content, degree of saturation with respect to hydroxy- and fluorapatite as well as change of surface microhardness (Knoop SMH) after 3 and 20 min incubation in different beverages and foodstuffs [in part from 47]

	pH	mmol OH⁻/l to pH 7.0	P_i (mmol/l)	Ca (mmol/l)	Fluoride (ppm)	pK–pI HAP	pK–pI FAP	Change in SMH after 3 min	Change in SMH after 20 min
Beverages (nonalcoholic)									
Citro light	3.0	75.0	<0.01	3.2	0.08	−25.7	−19.4		−103
Coca Cola	2.6	34.0	5.4	0.8	0.13	−19.2	−12.6	−136	−77
Fanta orange	2.9	83.6	0.1	0.8	0.05	−22.2	−16.1		−78
Ice tea	3.0	26.4	0.1	0.6	0.83	−22.3	−15.0	−107	−224
Isostar	3.8	34.0	1.6	1.8	0.14	−10.2	−4.2		−86
Isostar orange	3.6	31.4	3.4	5.8	0.18	−8.9	−2.6		−29
Aproz mineral water (sparklet)	5.3	24.0	<0.01	10.8	0.11	−5.8	−1.3		+6
Valser mineral water (sparklet)	5.4	34.6	0.01	10	0.58	−3.0	2.1	+8	+5
Valser lemon mineral water (sparklet)	3.3	68.0	<0.01	10.9	0.63	−17.2	−10.2	−54	−201
Orangina	3.2	70.0	0.4	0.4	0.07	−19.7	−13.6		−134
Pepsi light	3.1	34.6	3.9	0.9	0.04	−15.9	−9.8		−65
Perform	3.9	34.0	5.9	1.1	0.16	−9.2	−3.2		−6
Red Bull	3.4	91.6	<0.01	1.7	0.36	−19.8	−13.1	−123	−232
Sinalco	2.9	56.6	0.1	0.3	0.03	−23.7	−17.8		−110
Schweppes	2.5	88.6	<0.01	0.2	0.03	−32.8	−26.8		−136
Sprite	2.64	36.2	<0.01	0.2	0.04	−33.4	−27.3	−140	
Sprite light	2.9	62.0	<0.01	0.3	0.06	−30.5	−24.3		−162
Vitamin C effervescent tablet	3.98	105.4	<0.1	<0.1	0.03	−16.5	−11.3	−106	
Beverages (alcoholic)									
Carlsberg beer	4.4	40.0	7.3	2.2	0.28	−3.8	2.0		+8
Corona beer	4.2	8.2	3.3	2.1	0.11	−6.4	−0.8		+2
Hooch lemon	2.8	67.2	0.4	1.2	0.18	−19.8	−13.1		−257
Red wine	3.4	76.6	3.2	1.9	0.16	−12.3	−5.9		−71
White wine	3.7	70.0	3.2	0.9	0.35	−11.5	−5.0		−30

	pH	mmol OH⁻/l to pH 7.0	P_i (mmol/l)	Ca (mmol/l)	Fluoride (ppm)	pK-pl HAP	pK-pl FAP	Change in SMH after 3 min	Change in SMH after 20 min
Fruit juices									
Apple juice	3.4	82.0	1.7	4.0	0.11	−11.4	−5.2	−134	−154
Pineapple juice	3.43	60	1.9	1.7	0.04	−12.9	−7.2	−71	
Apple sauce	3.4	88.8	3.1	1.5	0.03	−13.2	−7.5		−186
Beetroot juice	4.2	49.2	10.0	2.1	0.08	−5.4	0.1	−40	−81
Carrot juice	4.2	42.0	8.4	5.0	0.09	−3.5	1.9	−5	−58
Grapefruit juice	3.2	218.0	2.6	3.1	0.16	−13.3	−6.8		−120
Grapefruit juice fresh squeezed	3.1	70.6	0.2	3.5	0.08	−16.4	−10.1		−109
Kiwi juice fresh squeezed	3.6	147.2	5.3	4.2	0.06	−9.2	−3.3	−102	−164
Multivitamin juice	3.6	131.4	6.5	4.8	0.12	−8.7	−2.5	−84	−137
Orange juice fresh	3.64	135.6	5.7	2.1	0.03	−9.7	−4.2	−115	
Orange juice	3.7	109.4	5.5	2.2	0.03	−9.4	−3.9	−26	−81
Milk products									
Milk	7.0	4.0	18.9	29.5	0.01	16.3	18.1		+11
Drinking whey	4.7	32.0	9.7	6.0	0.05	0.1	4.9		+1
Sour milk	4.2	56.0	39.2	69.0	0.03	2.4	7.4		+9
Yoghurt, natural	4.2	105.6	49.8	32.8	0.03	1.4	6.3	+1	+15
Yoghurt, kiwi	4.1	99.6	34.0	42.5	0.06	0.7	6.0	+4	+18
Yoghurt, lemon	4.1	110.4	39.9	32.0	0.04	0.4	5.6		+8
Yoghurt, orange	4.2	91.0	43.0	31.6	0.05	0.3	5.6	+1	
Yoghurt drink, orange	4.25	68.6	43.0	21.2	0.05	0.8	6.0	−1	
Probioplus yoghurt	4.26	81.6	47.2	27.6	0.03	1.4	6.4	+5	
Miscellaneous									
Rhubarb puree	2.77	344.8	7.75	12.974	0.4	−12.4	−5.3	−47	−62
Salad dressing	3.6	210.0	1.6	0.3	0.14	−15.6	−9.3		−109
Vinegar	3.2	740.8	2.2	3.4	1.20	−13.4	−6.0		−303

experiment (table 3). Many of the herbal teas were found to be even more erosive than orange juice [39]. In contrast to that, the milk products were all supersaturated with respect to both minerals and did not cause any softening of the surface after immersion of enamel in the respective products. Some flavored mineral water has in contrast to plain mineral water an erosive potential (table 3). This has some implication concerning the tooth health because the public is not aware of the erosive potential of these acidic drinks labeled as mineral water.

Fluoride present in the mouth during the daily de- and remineralization cycles gives rise to the formation of fluorapatite or fluorhydroxyapatite, which have a lower solubility than hydroxyapatite. Many of the acidic beverages or foodstuffs have a composition and a pH such that they are undersaturated with respect to these minerals and consequently even the outermost layer consisting of fluor(hydroxy)apatite will dissolve. Therefore, the protective effect of this outermost fluoride-rich mineral in preventing erosion is less important than it is in preventing caries. However, treatment with fluoride varnish (2.26%) for 24 h and high concentration F rinses (1.2%) for 48 h applied prior to acidic challenge have been shown to offer in vitro protection against erosion [11]. It is assumed that this protection is due to precipitation of calcium fluoride-like particles adhering to tooth surfaces which subsequently released fluoride over time. Hence, gentle fluoride application (without destruction of the protective acquired pellicle) before the erosive challenge would be most beneficial. The formation of the CaF_2-like layer on the tooth surface would act as a 'barrier' against acid attacks. This layer provides some additional mineral to be dissolved during an acid attack before the underlying enamel is attacked [40]. It is still controversial if these particles can be formed on sound tooth surface in vivo and in reasonable time. It has, however, been shown in vitro that KOH-soluble fluoride globules precipitate within a short time and in a higher amount when a low pH fluoride solution is used [41, 42]. The study by Larsen and Richards [41] further showed a beneficial effect of saliva on the formation of calcium fluoride-like material. Both a low pH of a fluoride solution with some subsequent loss of mineral and the calcium-rich saliva seem to be important factors in providing the system with calcium. It follows that deduction of a ranking for the in vivo erosivity of different acidic food and drinks based on pH, titratable acidity, Ca, P and F is rather complicated if not impossible. Besides these chemical factors, behavioral factors (such as eating and drinking habits, diets high in acidic fruits and vegetables, excessive consumption of acidic foods and drinks, oral hygiene practices) and biological factors (such as saliva flow rate, buffering capacity, acquired pellicle, dental anatomy and anatomy of oral soft tissues, physiological soft tissue movements) also have to be taken into account.

The adhesiveness and displacement of the liquid are other factors to be considered in the erosive process. There appear to be differences in the ability of beverages to adhere to enamel based on their thermodynamic properties, e.g. the thermodynamic work of adhesion [43]. The greater the adherence of an acidic substance is, the longer the contact time with the tooth surface and the higher the likelihood of erosion will be. It has been shown that displacement of saliva by Cola required $14\,mJ/m^2$, by Diet Cola $5\,mJ/m^2$. However, displacement of Cola film by saliva required $45\,mJ/m^2$, of Diet Cola by saliva $52\,mJ/m^2$. It seems to be more difficult to displace a soft drink film by saliva than it is to displace a salivary film by a soft drink [44]. Further research is needed to quantify the impact of all these factors in more detail. This has to be done by using reproducible and standardized methods. Guidelines on the testing of the erosive potential of foods derived from an international workshop were edited by Curzon and Hefferren [45].

In summary, it has been shown that the two very-often-cited parameters, pH and the titratable acidity, do not readily explain the erosive potential of food and drink. The mineral content is also an important parameter, as is the ability of any of the components to complex or chelate calcium and remove it from the mineral surface. Besides, these chemical factors several others such as the components of saliva and the flow rate of saliva have an impact on dental erosion in vivo. The degree of saturation with respect to the tooth mineral, hydroxyapatite and fluorapatite also strongly influence the erosion outcome. All of the above have to be taken into account to explain or even predict to some extent the influence of foods and beverages on dental hard tissue. Further, there is no clear-cut critical pH for erosion below which erosion will occur. Even at a low pH it is possible that other factors are strong enough to prevent erosion. At higher pH, it is possible that chemicals that complex calcium can cause erosion. The influence of all the factors described above in the fluid layer immediately in contact with the tooth surface determines whether erosion can proceed or not.

References

1   Miller WD: Experiments and observations on the wasting of tooth tissue erroneously designated as erosion, abrasion, denudation, etc. Dent Codmos 1907;49:109–124.
2   Restarski JS, Gortner RA, McCay CM: Effect of acid beverages containing fluorides upon the teeth of rats and puppies. J Am Dent Assoc 1945;32:668–675.
3   Miller CD: Enamel erosive properties of fruits and various beverages. J Am Diet Assoc 1952;28: 319–324.
4   Holloway PJ, Mellanby M, Stewart RJC: Fruit drinks and tooth erosion. Br Dent J 1958;104:305–309.
5   Stephan RM: Effects of different types of human foods on dental health in experimental animals. J Dent Res 1966;45:1551–1561.
6   Rytömaa I, Meurman JH, Koskinen J, Laakso T, Gharazi L, Turunen R: In vitro erosion of bovine enamel caused by acidic drinks and other foodstuffs. Scand J Dent Res 1988;96:324–333.

7   Beiraghi S, Atkins S, Rosen S, Wilson S, Odom J, Beck M: Effect of calcium lactate in erosion and *S. mutans* in rats when added to Coca-Cola. Pediatr Dent 1989;11:312–315.

8   Meurman JH, Härkönen M, Näveri H, Koskinen J, Torkko H, Rytömaa I, Järvinen V, Turunen R: Experimental sports drinks with minimal dental erosion effect. Scand J Dent Res 1990;98: 120–128.

9   Lussi A, Jaeggi T, Schärer S: The influence of different factors on in vitro enamel erosion. Caries Res 1993;27:387–393.

10 Mistry M, Grenby TH: Erosion by soft drinks of rat molar teeth assessed by digital image analysis. Caries Res 1993;27:21–25.

11 Sorvari R, Meurman JH, Alakuijala P, Frank RM: Effect of fluoride varnish and solution on enamel erosion in vitro. Caries Res 1994;28:227–232.

12 Grando LJ, Tames DR, Carsoso AC, Gabilan NH: In vitro study of enamel erosion caused by soft drinks and lemon juice in deciduous teeth analyzed by stereomicroscopy and scanning electron microscopy. Caries Res 1996;30:373–378.

13 Sorvari R, Pelttari A, Meurman JH: Surface ultrastructure of rat molar teeth after experimentally induced erosion and attrition. Caries Res 1996;30:163–168.

14 Maupomé G, Diez-de-Bonilla J, Torres-Villasenor G, Andrade-Delgado L, Castano VM: In vitro quantitative assessment of enamel microhardness after exposure to eroding immersion in cola drink. Caries Res 1998;32:148–153.

15 Meurman JH, ten Cate JM: Pathogenesis and modifying factors of dental erosion. Eur J Oral Sci 1996;104:199–206.

16 Grenby TH: Lessening dental erosive potential by product modification. Eur J Oral Sci 1996;104:221–228.

17 West NX, Hughes JA, Addy M: The effect of pH on the erosion of dentine and enamel by dietary acids in vitro. J Oral Rehabil 2001;28:860–864.

18 Hannig C, Hamkens A, Becker K, Attin R, Attin T: Erosive effects of different acids on bovine enamel: release of calcium and phosphate in vitro. Arch Oral Biol 2005;50:541–552.

19 Cairns AM, Watson M, Creanor SL, Foye RH: The pH and titratable acidity of a range of diluting drinks and their potential effect on dental erosion. J Dent 2002;30:313–317.

20 Lussi A, Jaeggi T, Jaeggi-Schärer S: Prediction of the erosive potential of some beverages. Caries Res 1995;29:349–354.

21 Larsen MJ: Dissolution of enamel. Scand J Dent Res 1973;81:518–522.

22 Larsen MJ, Nyvad B: Enamel erosion by some soft drinks and orange juices relative to their pH, buffering effect and contents of calcium phosphate. Caries Res 1999;33:81–87.

23 Barbour ME, Parker DM, Allen GC, Jandt KD: Human enamel erosion in constant composition citric acid solutions as a function of degree of saturation with respect to hydroxyapatite. J Oral Rehabil 2005;32:16–21.

24 Attin T, Meyer K, Hellwig E, Buchalla W, Lennon AM: Effect of mineral supplements to citric acid on enamel erosion. Arch Oral Biol 2003;48:753–759.

25 Attin T, Weiss K, Becker K, Buchalla W, Wiegand A: Impact of modified acidic soft drinks on enamel erosion. Oral Dis 2005;11:7–12.

26 Hughes JA, West NX, Parker DM, Newcombe RG, Addy M: Development and evaluation of a low erosive blackcurrant juice drink. 3. Final drink and concentrate, formulae comparison in situ and overview of the concept. J Dent 1999;27:345–350.

27 West NX, Hughes JA, Parker DM, Moohan M, Addy M: Development of low erosive carbonated blackcurrant drink compared to a conventional carbonated drink. J Dent 2003;31:361–365.

28 Hooper S, Hughes JA, Newcombe RG, Addy M, West NX: A methodology for testing the erosive potential of sports drinks. J Dent 2005;33:343–348.

29 Venables MC, Shaw L, Jeukendrup AE, Roedig-Penman A, Finke M, Newcombe RG, Parry J, Smith AJ: Erosive effect of a new sports drink on dental enamel during exercise. Med Sci Sports Exerc 2005;37:39–44.

30 Hooper S, West NX, Sharif N, Smith S, North M, De'Ath J, Parker DM, Roedig-Penman A, Addy M: A comparison of enamel erosion by a new sports drink compared to two proprietary products: a controlled, crossover study in situ. J Dent 2004;32:541–545.

31   Ramalingam L, Messer LB, Reynolds EC: Adding case in phosphopeptide-amorphous calcium phosphate to sports drinks to eliminate in vitro erosion. Pediatr Dent 2005;27:61–67.

32   Barbour ME, Parker DM, Allen GC, Jandt KD: Human enamel dissolution in citric acid as a function of pH in the range $2.30 \leq pH \leq 6.30$: a nanoindentation study. Eur J Oral Sci 2003;111:258–262.

33   Larsen MJ, Richards A: Fluoride is unable to reduce dental erosion from soft drinks. Caries Res 2002;36:75–80.

34   Mahoney E, Beattie J, Swain M, Kilpatrick N: Preliminary in vitro assessment of erosive potential using the ultra-micro-indentation system. Caries Res 2003;37:218–224.

35   Ganss C, Klimek J, Starck C: Quantitative analysis of the impact of the organic matrix on the fluoride effect on erosion progression in human dentine using longitudinal microradiography. Arch Oral Biol 2004;49:931–935.

36   Larsen MJ: An investigation of the theoretical background for the stability of the calcium phosphate salts and their mutual conversion in aqueous solutions. Arch Oral Biol 1986;31:757–761.

37   McDowell H, Gregory TM, Brown E: Solubility of $Ca_5(PO_4)_3OH$ in the system $Ca(OH)_2$-H_3PO_4-H_2O at 5, 15, 25 and 37°C. J Res Natl Bur Stand 1977;81A:273–281.

38   McCann HG: The solubility of fluorapatite and its relationship to that of calcium fluoride. Arch Oral Biol 1968;13:987–1001.

39   Phelan J, Rees J: The erosive potential of some herbal teas. J Dent 2003;31:241–246.

40   Ganss C, Klimek J, Schäfer U, Spall T: Effectiveness of two fluoridation measures on erosion progression in human enamel and dentine in vitro. Caries Res 2001;35:325–330.

41   Larsen MJ, Richards A: The influence of saliva on the formation of calcium fluoride-like material on human dental enamel. Caries Res 2001;35:57–60.

42   Petzold M: The influence of different fluoride compounds and treatment conditions on dental enamel: a descriptive in vitro study of the CaF_2 precipitation and microstructure. Caries Res 2001;35(suppl 1):45–51.

43   Ireland AJ, McGuinness N, Sherriff M: An investigation into the ability of soft drinks to adhere to enamel. Caries Res 1995;29:470–476.

44   Busscher HJ, Goedhart W, Ruben J, Bos R, Van der Mei CH: Wettability of dental enamel by soft drinks as compared to saliva and enamel demineralization; in Addy M, Embery G, Edgar WM, Orchardson R (eds): Tooth Wear and Sensitivity. London, Martin Dunitz, 2000, pp 197–200.

45   Curzon MEJ, Hefferren JJ: Modern methods for assessing the cariogenic and erosive potential of foods. Br Dent J 2001;191:41–46.

46   Zero D, Lussi A: Erosion: chemical and biological factors of importance to the dental practitioner. Int Dent J 2005;55:285–290.

47   Lussi A, Jaeggi T, Zero D: The role of diet in the aetiology of dental erosion. Caries Res 2004;38:34–44.

Prof. Dr. Adrian Lussi
Department of Preventive, Restorative and Pediatric Dentistry
School of Dental Medicine
University of Bern, Freiburgstrasse 7
CH–3010 Bern (Switzerland)

Lussi A (ed): Dental Erosion.
Monogr Oral Sci. Basel, Karger, 2006, vol 20, pp 88–99

....

Biological Factors

Anderson T. Hara[a], Adrian Lussi[b], Domenick T. Zero[a]

[a]Department of Preventive and Community Dentistry, Indiana University School of Dentistry, Indianapolis, Ind., USA; [b]Department of Preventive, Restorative and Pediatric Dentistry, School of Dental Medicine, University of Bern, Bern, Switzerland

Abstract

Biological factors such as saliva, acquired dental pellicle, tooth structure and positioning in relation to soft tissues and tongue are related to dental erosion development. Saliva has been shown to be the most important biological factor in the prevention of dental erosion. It starts acting even before the acid attack, with the increase of the salivary flow rate as a response to the acidic stimuli. This creates a favorable scenario, increasing the buffering system of saliva and effectively diluting and clearing acids on dental surfaces during the erosive challenge. Saliva plays a role in the formation of the acquired dental pellicle, which acts as a perm-selective membrane preventing contact of the acid with the tooth surfaces. The protective level of the pellicle seems to be regulated by its composition, thickness and maturation time. Due to its mineral content, saliva can also prevent demineralization as well as enhance remineralization. However, these preventive and reparative factors of saliva may not be enough against highly erosive challenges, leading to erosion development. The progress rate of erosion can be significantly influenced by the type of dental substrate, occurrence of mechanical and chemical attacks, fluoride exposure, and also by contact with the oral soft tissues and tongue.

The biological factors related to dental erosion may involve properties and characteristics of saliva, acquired dental pellicle, tooth structure and surrounding soft tissues [1, 2]. The interaction of these factors with both erosive agent and behavioral aspects, over time, may influence the development as well as the prevention, arrest and possibly recovery of erosive lesions [3]. A critical review based on clinical and laboratorial findings will follow in an attempt to clarify the impact of the biological factors on the dental erosion process.

Saliva

Saliva has been considered the most important biological factor influencing dental erosion prevention due to its ability to act, directly on the erosive agent itself by diluting, clearing, neutralizing and buffering acids, play a role in forming a protective membrane, and to reduce the demineralization rate and enhance remineralization by providing calcium, phosphate and fluoride to eroded enamel and dentin. The relevance of saliva on the erosion process could be better illustrated by a comparison between in vitro – with no salivary protection – and in situ erosion models, where it was shown that enamel erosion was dramatically reduced by the order of 10 times in the in situ model [4].

Saliva starts its protective effect against erosion even before the acid challenge, by the increase of the flow rate as a response to the extra-oral stimuli such as odor [5, 6] or sight [7]. Studies have shown that sour foodstuff has a strong influence on the anticipatory salivary flow [5, 7], which can be significantly increased when compared to the normal unstimulated flow rate [6]. Hypersalivation also occurs in advance of vomiting as a response from the 'vomiting center' of the brain [8], as frequently seen in individuals suffering from anorexia and bulimia nervosa, rumination or chronic alcoholism. It is suggested that this could minimize the erosion caused by acids of gastric origin. On the other hand, patients with symptoms of gastro-esophageal reflux disease should not expect the salivary output to increase before the gastric juice regurgitation, because this is an involuntary response not co-coordinated by the autonomic nervous system [9]. Therefore, there may be insufficient time for saliva to act before erosion occurs.

Higher salivary flow rate creates a favorably scenario for the prevention or minimization of initial erosive attack due to the increase of the organic and inorganic constituents of saliva. The inorganic constituents of primary interest in the erosion process are carbonic acid (H_2CO_3)/hydrogen carbonate (HCO_3^-), di-hydrogenphosphate ($H_2PO_4^-$)/hydrogen phosphate (HPO_4^{2-}), calcium (Ca^{2+}) and fluoride (F^-) [10, 11]. These ions are associated with enhancing the buffer capacity of saliva and maintenance of the integrity of teeth [12]. Hydrogen carbonate is the principal buffer of saliva and its concentration increases from about 5 mmol/l in unstimulated up to 60 mmol/l in stimulated whole saliva. The concentration of di-hydrogenphosphate is regulated in the opposite direction from 5 mmol/l unstimulated saliva down to 3 mmol/l in stimulated saliva [13]. The protein buffer system may also be of some importance in lower pH levels (below 4.5). Acidic proline-rich proteins, found in parotid saliva, as well as mucins, the major organic component of submandibular/sublingual saliva, are important constituents of the acquired pellicle and plaque matrix [14, 15]. Mucins can also reduce the abrasive wear of eroded areas since they present lubrication properties [14].

Once the acid reaches the mouth several mechanisms of saliva come into play to protect the teeth. Intra-oral stimuli of the salivary flow are mainly due to chemical and mechanical stimulation. Potentially erosive foodstuff and beverages, such those with citric or malic acid content [16], elicit a strong response. Three droplets of 4% citric acid applied to the tongue every 30 s for 5 min caused the mean flow rate to rise up to about 1.87 ml/min, which was significantly higher when compared to the unstimulated flow of about 0.38 ml/min [6]. Mastication can also stimulate the saliva output [17]. It has been suggested that the stimulation of the mechanoreceptive neurons in the gingival tissues may result in a reflex secretion of saliva [18]. Depending on the oral stimuli, different salivary glands may be affected leading to the variation in salivary flow and composition [6], thus influencing the level of salivary protection.

A higher flow rate with higher hydrogen bicarbonate content increases the capacity of saliva in neutralizing and buffering acids as well as the ability to clear acids on teeth surfaces, as shown in previous studies [19–22]. Even though acid clearance has been reported as an individual property [23], it can be suggested that factors such as food consistency and sites of the mouth affect the acid clearance pattern. Sites poorly bathed by saliva or mainly bathed with mucous saliva are more likely to show erosion when compared to sites protected by serous saliva [24, 25]. Thus, the facial surfaces of upper incisors would be more prone to erosion and the opposite is true for the lingual surfaces of lower teeth [25]. The time required for saliva to neutralize and/or clear the acid from the tooth surface has been measured in vivo with pH electrodes, and it has shown to range between 2 and 5 min [26]. Bartlett et al. [27] reported similar ranges of 3 and 7 min, but also reported a wide variance, suggesting that the buffering and clearance capacities are strongly related to individual variations.

The impact of erosion in patients suffering from salivary flow impairment can clearly demonstrate the importance of saliva. Studies have shown that erosion is strongly associated with low salivary flow and low buffering capacity [19, 20, 28, 29]. The dry mouth condition is usually related to aging [11, 30, 31], even though some other studies have not found this correlation [32, 33]. It is well-established that patients taking medication can also present decreased saliva output [34], as well as those who have received radiation therapy for neck and head cancer [35]. Tests of the stimulated and unstimulated flow rate as well as of the buffer capacity of saliva may provide useful information about the susceptibility of an individual to dental erosion. Sialometric evaluations should be carried at a fixed time-point or in a limited time interval in the morning, avoiding intra-individual variations due to the circadian cycle [36].

Acquired Dental Salivary Pellicle

The salivary acquired pellicle is a protein-based layer which is rapidly formed on dental surfaces after its removal by tooth brushing with dentifrice, chemical dissolution or prophylaxis. This organic layer becomes detectable on dental surfaces after few minutes of exposure to the oral environment, as previously shown by electron microscopy analyses [37, 38]. Biological, i.e. enzymatic, activity is also detectable on early stages of pellicle formation [39, 40]. It is suggested that it grows until reaching an equilibrium between protein adsorption and de-sorption within 2 h [41]. As described by Skjorland et al. [37], pellicle formation appears to involve a two-step process. In the first step, initial adsorption of discrete proteins is thought to occur by electrostatic interactions with the hydrophobic regions of the tooth, leaving hydrophobic parts of the protein molecules exposed at the surface. Either as a second step or as an independent process, protein aggregates or micelle-like structures may adsorb to uncovered sites on the tooth surface and also interact with the initially formed hydrophobic protein layer [37, 42]. This specific adsorption pattern may be responsible for the globular morphology of the acquired pellicle, as previously described [43, 44].

The acquired pellicle may protect against erosion by acting as a diffusion barrier or a perm-selective membrane preventing the direct contact between the acids and the tooth surface [38, 45, 46], reducing the dissolution rate of hydroxyapatite [41]. This protective effect could be clearly visualized by a scanning electron microscopy study, where the 2-h formed pellicle was able to reduce erosion by an acidic beverage [47]. This protection on enamel surfaces has also been quantified by in vitro and in situ studies. Nekrashevych and Stösser [48] showed that 24-h pellicles formed in vitro were able to totally or partially prevent enamel surface microhardness change resulting from a 1-min exposure to 0.1% citric acid or 5 min exposure to 1% citric acid, respectively. Hannig and Balz [49], in an in situ investigation, found that a 24-h formed pellicle can show some protection against acid challenge performed by 0.1–1% citric acid for up to 5 min. Amaechi et al. [50] showed that 1-h acquired pellicle formed in situ could protect enamel against demineralization from 2 h of in vitro orange juice exposure.

Although it seems to be clear that pellicle can interfere in the demineralization of the dental surfaces by erosive acids, the composition, thickness and maturation time of the pellicle may significantly define the protection level against dental erosion. The dental pellicle can serve as a reservoir of remineralizing electrolytes [40], which might influence erosion development. In vitro studies have shown that salivary mucins of the pellicle have the capacity to increase enamel surface protection against demineralization [14]. However, Hannig and

Balz [43] could not find differences in the protective level of an in situ-formed pellicle with different mucin concentrations. The presence of the salivary enzyme carbonic anhydrase VI in pellicle may protect against dental erosion, by accelerating the neutralization of hydrogen ions on the tooth surface [40].

Differences in the site of pellicle formation in the mouth contribute to the thickness of the pellicle, which in turn influence the level of protection against enamel demineralization. An in situ study showed that the thinnest pellicles (about 0.3–0.38 μm) were formed on the palatal surface of upper teeth, while the thickest pellicles (about 0.96–1.06 μm) were formed on lingual surfaces after 1 h of intra-oral exposure [50]. In agreement with these findings, Hannig and Balz [43] reported that 24-h pellicle formed in situ on specimens positioned at the palate [49] tended to be thinner and less resistant to the citric acid treatment than the lingually and buccally formed pellicles. These data may partially support the results of a clinical study of the prevalence of erosive lesions [25]. This study reported that the sites of greater pellicle thickness (lingual surfaces) showed lower percentage of erosion (about 1.7–2%). However, they also found that sites thought to be covered by a thinner pellicle (palatal surfaces) also showed lower percentages (2.7–6.1%) of erosion. This can be explained by the higher salivary clearance expected for the palatal surfaces [25], as discussed before.

Although the pellicle may reach its full thickness within 2 h, some structural modification may happen after this period as part of the maturation process of the freshly formed pellicle causing it to become more acid-resistant. It has been suggested by in vitro studies that this process of the pellicle may increase the protection of the pellicle as a diffusion barrier to ionic conductivity on enamel surface [14, 51–53]. This was suggested to take 18 h in vivo and at least 4 days in vitro. According to Lendenmann et al. [41], this difference is due to enzymes, possibly transglutaminase [54, 55] that is continuously re-supplied in the mouth but rapidly loses its activity in vitro due to a short half-life. Enzymes are assumed to have influence on the structural remodeling of the acquired pellicle during the maturation process in vivo [40, 56] and could be necessary for stabilizing and creating a more acid-resistant pellicle [41].

Much has been discussed and is expected to be discovered about the composition and maturation process of the pellicle on its ability to prevent erosion. This information is essential not only to understand the protective mechanism of the pellicle but also to estimate how protective the pellicle can be against erosive challenges of different aggressiveness. As stated above, it has been proved that pellicles of different compositions and maturation levels protect against erosion but some studies have highlighted that it is not a complete inhibition [39]. Hara et al. [57] showed that a 2-h acquired pellicle formed on enamel surfaces in situ was able to reduce the demineralization provided by orange juice up to 10 min of acid exposure (fig. 1a, b), using the in situ erosion model

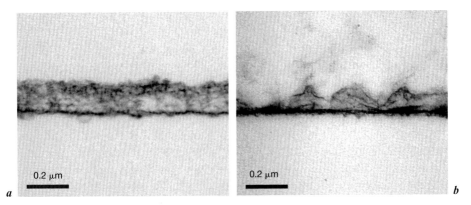

a

b

Fig. 1. *a* Transmission electron microscopy image of the 2-h in situ formed pellicle on enamel surface. *b* The 2-h pellicle after 10 min of erosive challenge in situ by orange juice. Even after partial dissolution, the pellicle was still able to provide some protection to enamel.

previously reported by Zero et al. [58]. However, no measurable protection was detected after 20 and 30 min of acid exposure. It was speculated that the 10-min acid exposure, which consisted of sipping 10 ml of the juice, holding it for 15 s in the mouth, spiting and resting for 15 s to repeat the procedure for 39 more times, could simulate the ingestion of a regular cup of beverage (400 ml) over a 20-min period. This level of acid exposure is considered a high risk of erosion behavior. Interestingly, no protection could be found in this study for the dentin substrate covered by the 2-h pellicle. At this point there is no adequate information to support that it was due to differences in the pellicles composition, but it has been suggested that differences in the substrates' nature and composition may affect the pellicle composition and properties [59]. It could also be suggested that no protection was found for dentin because of the higher susceptibility of dentin to demineralization, which could have resulted in the pellicle being lost together with the etched dentin [57].

As it has been shown, the salivary protection against erosion may not be enough to prevent erosion. These above-mentioned biological factors are best understood if considered as a physiologic host response to occasional or mild episodes of acid challenge in the mouth. No pathological consequences occur unless the acid challenge (strength and/or frequency) exceeds a certain threshold or the host response is not adequate to counteract the erosive challenge. As emphasized by Meurman et al. [20], if the erosive challenge is strong enough even normal salivary flow and function cannot protect the teeth. As a consequence, dental erosion could be dramatically enhanced by highly erosive challenges and/or by salivary diseases. The response of the tooth structure to these attacks should also be taken into consideration.

Biological Factors

Tooth Structure

Enamel is the most at risk surface for erosion and thus has received the most attention. More recently, dentin has also been considered. Since teeth are being kept in the mouth for longer, exposure of coronal dentin as well as of root dentin is becoming clinically common as a result of tooth wear and gingival recession, respectively.

The process of enamel erosion involves an initial softening of the surface followed by permanent loss of the demineralized tooth structure due to the erosive attack by acids [60]. In dentin, the inorganic content can be etched away with the erosive attack; however, the organic content is thought to remain. The exposed organic content of dentin may act as a barrier either to the acid diffusion or to the mineral release, thus reducing the lesion progression [61, 62]. For this reason, the chemical or mechanical removal of the organic material may significantly accelerate the rate of lesion progression [62] and prevent a possible mineral deposition on the eroded area to occur [63].

The above-mentioned processes have been described for sound enamel and dentin. Although, they are valuable and essential to the understanding of the erosion progress, it should be considered that in clinical situations different lesion progress patterns may occur since the tooth substrate can be previously affected by chemical and mechanical factors (e.g. caries, erosion, abrasion, fluorosis). The susceptibility to erosion in such conditions is not well known and deserves further research. The influence of fluoride as fluoridated apatite or CaF_2-like particles in the erosion progress is discussed in details in a specific chapter of this book.

Exposure to saliva, dietary products and fluoride has been shown to be effective in the remineralization of eroded enamel. Once the erosive agent is neutralized or cleared from the tooth surface, the deposition of salivary calcium and phosphate can lead to remineralization of softened enamel [64–66]. The effect of the remineralization time has also been investigated [22]. Enamel specimens eroded by citric acid for 2 h and immersed in artificial saliva showed partial rehardening after 1–4 h, while specimens remineralized for 6–24 h showed a complete rehardening. An in situ study, analyzing the surface microhardness recovery of enamel and dentin eroded by acidic beverage, showed up to 37.8% of remineralization of enamel specimens, after 24 h of exposure to the oral environment [67]. When treated with fluoride gel after the erosive attack, the remineralization rate of enamel specimens significantly increased to 57.2%. Similarly, it was shown that eroded dentin had a surface microhardness recovery of about 55.4%; however, there was no significant increase related to treatment with fluoride gel [67].

Recently, given the increasing attention to esthetic dental procedures, dental bleaching has been investigated for possible detrimental side effects on

Table 1. Biological factors influencing the erosive tooth wear

• Saliva: flow rate, composition, buffering capacity and stimulation capacity
• Acquired pellicle: diffusion-limiting properties, composition, maturation and thickness
• Type of dental substrate (permanent and primary enamel, dentin) and composition (e.g. fluoride content as FHAP or CaF_2-like particles)
• Dental anatomy and occlusion
• Anatomy of oral soft tissues in relationship to the teeth
• Physiological soft tissue movements

enamel and dentin. It has been shown that some hydrogen peroxide-based gels may influence enamel surface morphology [68, 69] and softening [70, 71] suggesting an increased susceptibility to dental erosion [72]. These changes are thought to be related to the specific experimental conditions used or to the properties of the products. Some of the studies did not include artificial or human saliva to simulate clinical conditions [69, 70, 73], while others that did have not shown the same damage to the enamel and dentin surfaces [74–77]. The concentration of hydrogen peroxide, the fluoride content and the pH of the bleaching agent are factors that may also be responsible for alterations of dental hard tissues [72, 77, 78]. Indeed, the use of bleaching agents with lower content of hydrogen peroxide and neutral pH did not increase the susceptibility of enamel to erosion in vitro [77].

Some controversy remains about the susceptibility of primary teeth compared to permanents. Differences in the mineralization level may render primary teeth to be one and a half times more susceptible to demineralization than permanent teeth [79]. However, it was also reported that there was no change in the susceptibility of these substrates to erosion when challenged by several acid beverages in an in vitro comparison [80]. Even though a higher prevalence of tooth wear has been shown for children when compared to adults, it might be due to the overlap of the erosive challenge with the abrasive procedures [81, 82], since the primary enamel is supposed to be less resistant to abrasion [80].

Dental Positioning and Soft Tissues

Different positioning of the teeth in the dental arch may provide different susceptibility of the tooth surface to erosion. As previously discussed, erosion is highly influenced by the protective factors of saliva, such as flow rate (clearance) and composition (buffering and remineralizing capacity), which vary in different sites of the mouth. Hence, the facial surfaces of upper incisors and lingual surfaces of lower teeth have, respectively, higher and lower susceptibility to erosion. Another significant aspect is the relationship of the teeth to the surrounding soft tissues and tongue. Holst and Lange [83] considered the abrasion caused by tongue to be a contributing factor in erosion caused by vomiting. It was showed by an in vitro investigation that tongue was able to remove enamel and dentin softened by erosion [84]. In agreement, an in situ study showed that unprotected eroded enamel was significant more susceptible to wear, by the contact with oral soft tissues and food, when compared to mechanically protected surfaces [85]. A similar effect was also suggested by another in situ study testing the surface wear of eroded dentin [86]. These studies corroborate the findings from a clinical trial by Järvinen et al. [87], where it was found that the most severe erosive lesions were located at the palatal surfaces of the upper teeth, suggesting the abrasive effect of the tongue. Other variables such as the relationship between the size of the tongue and the dental arches, as well as the positioning of the teeth may contribute to increasing the progression of erosion.

References

1   Zero DT: Etiology of dental erosion: extrinsic factors. Eur J Oral Sci 1996;104:162–177.
2   Lussi A, Jaeggi T, Zero D: The role of diet in the aetiology of dental erosion. Caries Res 2004;38: 34–44.
3   Zero DT, Lussi A: Etiology of enamel erosion: intrinsic and extrinsic factors; in Addy M, Embery G, Edgar WM, Orchardson R (eds): Tooth Wear and Sensitivity. London, Martin Dunitz, 2000, pp 121–139.
4   West NX, Maxwell A, Hughes JA, Parker DM, Newcombe RG, Addy M: A method to measure clinical erosion: the effect of orange juice consumption on erosion of enamel. J Dent 1998;26:329–335.
5   Lee VM, Linden RW: An olfactory-submandibular salivary reflex in humans. Exp Physiol 1992;77:221–224.
6   Engelen L, de Wijk RA, Prinz JF, van der Bilt A, Bosman F: The relation between saliva flow after different stimulations and the perception of flavor and texture attributes in custard desserts. Physiol Behav 2003;78:165–169.
7   Christensen CM, Navazesh M: Anticipatory salivary flow to the sight of different foods. Appetite 1984;5:307–315.
8   Lee M, Feldman M: Nausea and vomiting; in Feldman M, Scharschmidt B, Sleisenger M (eds): Sleisenger and Fordstran's Gastrointestinal and Liver Disease: Pathophysiology, Diagnosis, Management, ed 6. Philadelphia, Saunders, 1998, pp 117–127.
9   Saksena R, Bartlett DW, Smith BG: The role of saliva in regurgitation erosion. Eur J Prosthodont Restor Dent 1999;7:121–124.
10 Larsen MJ, Pearce EI: Saturation of human saliva with respect to calcium salts. Arch Oral Biol 2003;48:317–322.
11 Dodds MW, Johnson DA, Yeh CK: Health benefits of saliva: a review. J Dent 2005;33:223–233.
12 Dawes C, Kubieniec K: The effects of prolonged gum chewing on salivary flow rate and composition. Arch Oral Biol 2004;49:665–669.
13 Ferguson DB: Salivary glands and saliva; in Lavelle CLB (eds): Applied Physiology of the Mouth. Bristol, John Wright, 1975, pp 145–179.
14 Nieuw Amerongen AV, Oderkerk CH, Driessen AA: Role of mucins from human whole saliva in the protection of tooth enamel against demineralization in vitro. Caries Res 1987;21:297–309.
15 Schupbach P, Oppenheim FG, Lendenmann U, Lamkin MS, Yao Y, Guggenheim B: Electron-microscopic demonstration of proline-rich proteins, statherin, and histatins in acquired enamel pellicles in vitro. Eur J Oral Sci 2001;109:60–68.

16   Hay DI, Pinsent BRW, Schram CJ, Wagg BJ: The protective effect of calcium and phosphate ions against acid erosion of dental enamel and dentin. Br Dent J 1962;3:283–287.

17   Yeh CK, Johnson DA, Dodds MW, Sakai S, Rugh JD, Hatch JP: Association of salivary flow rates with maximal bite force. J Dent Res 2000;79:1560–1565.

18   Scott BJ, Bajaj J, Linden RW: The contribution of mechanoreceptive neurones in the gingival tissues to the masticatory-parotid salivary reflex in man. J Oral Rehabil 1999;26:791–797.

19   Jarvinen VK, Rytomaa II, Heinonen OP: Risk factors in dental erosion. J Dent Res 1991;70:942–947.

20   Meurman JH, Toskala J, Nuutinen P, Klemetti E: Oral and dental manifestations in gastroesophageal reflux disease. Oral Surg Oral Med Oral Pathol 1994;78:583–589.

21   Lussi A, Schaffner M: Progression of and risk factors for dental erosion and wedge-shaped defects over a 6-year period. Caries Res 2000;34:182–187.

22   Eisenburger M, Addy M, Hughes JA, Shellis RP: Effect of time on the remineralisation of enamel by synthetic saliva after citric acid erosion. Caries Res 2001;35:211–215.

23   Bashir E, Ekberg O, Lagerlof F: Salivary clearance of citric acid after an oral rinse. J Dent 1995;23: 209–212.

24   Dawes C: Physiological factors affecting salivary flow rate, oral sugar clearance, and the sensation of dry mouth in man. J Dent Res 1987;66:648–653.

25   Young WG, Khan F: Sites of dental erosion are saliva-dependent. J Oral Rehabil 2002;29:35–43.

26   Millward A, Shaw L, Harrington E, Smith AJ: Continuous monitoring of salivary flow rate and pH at the surface of the dentition following consumption of acidic beverages. Caries Res 1997;31: 44–49.

27   Bartlett DW, Bureau GP, Anggiansah A: Evaluation of the pH of a new carbonated soft drink beverage: an in vivo investigation. J Prosthodont 2003;12:21–25.

28   Bartlett DW, Coward PY, Nikkah C, Wilson RF: The prevalence of tooth wear in a cluster sample of adolescent schoolchildren and its relationship with potential explanatory factors. Br Dent J 1998;184:125–129.

29   Rytomaa I, Jarvinen V, Kanerva R, Heinonen OP: Bulimia and tooth erosion. Acta Odontol Scand 1998;56:36–40.

30   Percival RS, Challacombe SJ, Marsh PD: Flow rates of resting whole and stimulated parotid saliva in relation to age and gender. J Dent Res 1994;73:1416–1420.

31   Navazesh M, Mulligan RA, Kipnis V, Denny PA, Denny PC: Comparison of whole saliva flow rates and mucin concentrations in healthy Caucasian young and aged adults. J Dent Res 1992;71: 1275–1278.

32   Heintze U, Birkhed D, Bjorn H: Secretion rate and buffer effect of resting and stimulated whole saliva as a function of age and sex. Swed Dent J 1983;7:227–238.

33   Ben-Aryeh H, Shalev A, Szargel R, Laor A, Laufer D, Gutman D: The salivary flow rate and composition of whole and parotid resting and stimulated saliva in young and old healthy subjects. Biochem Med Metab Biol 1986;36:260–265.

34   Wynn RL, Meiller TF: Drugs and dry mouth. Gen Dent 2001;49:10–14.

35   Dreizen S, Brown LR, Daly TE, Drane JB: Prevention of xerostomia-related dental caries in irradiated cancer patients. J Dent Res 1977;56:99–104.

36   Flink H, Tegelberg A, Lagerlof F: Influence of the time of measurement of unstimulated human whole saliva on the diagnosis of hyposalivation. Arch Oral Biol 2005;50:553–559.

37   Skjorland KK, Rykke M, Sonju T: Rate of pellicle formation in vivo. Acta Odontol Scand 1995;53:358–362.

38   Hannig M: Ultrastructural investigation of pellicle morphogenesis at two different intraoral sites during a 24-h period. Clin Oral Investig 1999;3:88–95.

39   Hannig M, Fiebiger M, Guntzer M, Dobert A, Zimehl R, Nekrashevych Y: Protective effect of the in situ formed short-term salivary pellicle. Arch Oral Biol 2004;49:903–910.

40   Hannig C, Hannig M, Attin T: Enzymes in the acquired enamel pellicle. Eur J Oral Sci 2005;113: 2–13.

41   Lendenmann U, Grogan J, Oppenheim FG: Saliva and dental pellicle: a review. Adv Dent Res 2000;14:22–28.

42   Vitkov L, Hannig M, Nekrashevych Y, Krautgartner WD: Supramolecular pellicle precursors. Eur J Oral Sci 2004;112:320–325.

43   Rolla G, Rykke M: Evidence for the presence of micelle-like protein globules in human saliva. Colloids Surf 1994;3:177–182.

44   Hannig M, Balz M: Protective properties of salivary pellicles from two different intraoral sites on enamel erosion. Caries Res 2001;35:142–148.

45   Zahradnik RT, Propas D, Moreno EC: In vitro enamel demineralization by *Streptococcus mutans* in the presence of salivary pellicles. J Dent Res 1977;56:1107–1110.

46   Zahradnik RT, Propas D, Moreno EC: Effect of fluoride topical solutions on enamel demineralization by lactate buffers and *Streptococcus mutans* in vitro. J Dent Res 1978;57:940–946.

47   Meurman JH, Frank RM: Scanning electron microscopic study of the effect of salivary pellicle on enamel erosion. Caries Res 1991;25:1–6.

48   Nekrashevych Y, Stösser L: Protective influence of experimentally formed salivary pellicle on enamel erosion. An in vitro study. Caries Res 2003;37:225–231.

49   Hannig M, Balz M: Influence of in vivo formed salivary pellicle on enamel erosion. Caries Res 1999;33:372–379.

50   Amaechi BT, Higham SM, Edgar WM, Milosevic A: Thickness of acquired salivary pellicle as a determinant of the sites of dental erosion. J Dent Res 1999;78:1821–1828.

51   Featherstone JD, Behrman JM, Bell JE: Effect of whole saliva components on enamel demineralization in vitro. Crit Rev Oral Biol Med 1993;4:357–362.

52   Kautsky MB, Featherstone JD: Effect of salivary components on dissolution rates of carbonated apatites. Caries Res 1993;27:373–377.

53   Duschner H, Hermann G, Walker R, Lussi A: Erosion of dental enamel visualized by confocal laser scanning microscopy; in Addy M, Embery G, Edgar WM, Orchardson R (eds): Tooth Wear and Sensitivity. London, Martin Dunitz, 2000, pp 67–73.

54   Yao Y, Lamkin MS, Oppenheim FG: Pellicle precursor proteins: acidic proline-rich proteins, statherin, and histatins, and their crosslinking reaction by oral transglutaminase. J Dent Res 1999;78:1696–1703.

55   Yao Y, Lamkin MS, Oppenheim FG: Pellicle precursor protein crosslinking characterization of an adduct between acidic proline-rich protein (PRP-1) and statherin generated by transglutaminase. J Dent Res 2000;79:930–938.

56   Yao Y, Grogan J, Zehnder M, Lendenmann U, Nam B, Wu Z, Costello CE, Oppenheim FG: Compositional analysis of human acquired enamel pellicle by mass spectrometry. Arch Oral Biol 2001;46:293–303.

57   Hara AT, Ando M, González-Cabezas C, Cury JA, Serra MC, Zero DT: Protective effect of the acquired enamel pellicle against different erosive challenges in situ. Caries Res 2004;38:390.

58   Zero DT, Barillas I, Hayes AL, Fu J, Li H: Evaluation of an intraoral model for the study of dental erosion. Caries Res 1998;32:312.

59   Glantz PO, Baier RE, Christersson CE: Biochemical and physiological considerations for modeling biofilms in the oral cavity: a review. Dent Mater 1996;12:208–214.

60   Attin T, Koidl U, Buchalla W, Schaller HG, Kielbassa AM, Hellwig E: Correlation of microhardness and wear in differently eroded bovine dental enamel. Arch Oral Biol 1997;42:243–250.

61   Vanuspong W, Eisenburger M, Addy M: Cervical tooth wear and sensitivity: erosion, softening and rehardening of dentine: effects of pH, time and ultrasonication. J Clin Periodontol 2002;29:351–357.

62   Hara AT, Ando M, Cury JA, Serra MC, Gonzalez-Cabezas C, Zero DT: Influence of the organic matrix on root dentine erosion by citric acid. Caries Res 2005;39:134–138.

63   Ganss C, Klimek J, Brune V, Schurmann A: Effects of two fluoridation measures on erosion progression in human enamel and dentine in situ. Caries Res 2004;38:561–566.

64   Feagin F, Koulourides T, Pigman W: The characterization of enamel surface demineralization, remineralization, and associated hardness changes in human and bovine material. Arch Oral Biol 1969;14:1407–1417.

65   Gedalia I, Dakuar A, Shapira L, Lewinstein I, Goultschin J, Rahamim E: Enamel softening with Coca-Cola and rehardening with milk or saliva. Am J Dent 1991;4:120–122.

66   Zero DT, Fu J, Scott-Anne K, Proskin H: Evaluation of fluoride dentifrices using a short-term intraoral remineralization model. J Dent Res 1994;73:272.

67   Fushida CE, Cury JA: Evaluation of enamel-dentine erosion by beverage and recovery by saliva and fluoride. J Dent Res 1999;78:410.

68   Flaitz CM, Hicks MJ: Effects of carbamide peroxide whitening agents on enamel surfaces and caries-like lesion formation: an SEM and polarized light microscopic in vitro study. ASDC J Dent Child 1996;63:249–256.

69   Zalkind M, Arwaz JR, Goldman A, Rotstein I: Surface morphology changes in human enamel, dentin and cementum following bleaching: a scanning electron microscopy study. Endod Dent Traumatol 1996;12:82–88.

70   Murchison DF, Charlton DG, Moore BK: Carbamide peroxide bleaching: effects on enamel surface hardness and bonding. Oper Dent 1992;17:181–185.

71   Rodrigues JA, Basting RT, Serra MC, Rodrigues Junior AL: Effects of 10% carbamide peroxide bleaching materials on enamel microhardness. Am J Dent 2001;14:67–71.

72   Attin T, Kocabiyik M, Buchalla W, Hannig C, Becker K: Susceptibility of enamel surfaces to demineralization after application of fluoridated carbamide peroxide gels. Caries Res 2003;37:93–99.

73   Rotstein I, Dankner E, Goldman A, Heling I, Stabholz A, Zalkind M: Histochemical analysis of dental hard tissues following bleaching. J Endod 1996;22:23–25.

74   Basting RT, Rodrigues AL Jr, Serra MC: The effects of seven carbamide peroxide bleaching agents on enamel microhardness over time. J Am Dent Assoc 2003;134:1335–1342.

75   de Freitas PM, Turssi CP, Hara AT, Serra MC: Monitoring of demineralized dentin microhardness throughout and after bleaching. Am J Dent 2004;17:342–346.

76   Arcari GM, Baratieri LN, Maia HP, De Freitas SF: Influence of the duration of treatment using a 10% carbamide peroxide bleaching gel on dentin surface microhardness: an in situ study. Quintessence Int 2005;36:15–24.

77   Pretty IA, Edgar WM, Higham SM: The effect of bleaching on enamel susceptibility to acid erosion and demineralisation. Br Dent J 2005;198:285–290.

78   Frysh H, Bowles WH, Baker F, Rivera-Hidalgo F, Guillen G: Effect of pH on hydrogen peroxide bleaching agents. J Esthet Dent 1995;7:130–133.

79   Amaechi BT, Higham SM, Edgar WM: Factors influencing the development of dental erosion in vitro: enamel type, temperature and exposure time. J Oral Rehabil 1999;26:624–630.

80   Lussi A, Kohler N, Zero D, Schaffner M, Megert B: A comparison of the erosive potential of different beverages in primary and permanent teeth using an in vitro model. Eur J Oral Sci 2000;108:110–114.

81   Jones SG, Nunn JH: The dental health of 3-year-old children in east Cumbria 1993. Community Dent Health 1995;12:161–166.

82   Millward A, Shaw L, Smith AJ, Rippin JW, Harrington E: The distribution and severity of tooth wear and the relationship between erosion and dietary constituents in a group of children. Int J Paediatr Dent 1994;4:151–157.

83   Holst JJ, Lange F: Perimylolysis. A contribution towards the genesis of tooth wasting from non-mechanical causes. Acta Odontol Scand 1939;1:36–48.

84   Gregg T, Mace S, West NX, Addy M: A study in vitro of the abrasive effect of the tongue on enamel and dentine softened by acid erosion. Caries Res 2004;38:557–560.

85   Amaechi BT, Higham SM, Edgar WM: Influence of abrasion in clinical manifestation of human dental erosion. J Oral Rehabil 2003;30:407–413.

86   Hara AT, Turssi CP, Teixeira EC, Serra MC, Cury JA: Abrasive wear on eroded root dentine after different periods of exposure to saliva in situ. Eur J Oral Sci 2003;111:423–427.

87   Järvinen V, Rytomaa I, Meurman JH: Location of dental erosion in a referred population. Caries Res 1992;26:391–396.

Dr. Anderson T. Hara
Department of Preventive and Community
Dentistry, Indiana University
School of Dentistry
415 N. Lansing Street
Indianapolis, IN 46202-2876 (USA)

Lussi A (ed): Dental Erosion.
Monogr Oral Sci. Basel, Karger, 2006, vol 20, pp 100–105

······················

Behavioral Factors

D.T. Zero[a], *A. Lussi*[b]

[a]Department of Preventive and Community Dentistry, Indiana University School of Dentistry, Indianapolis, Ind., USA; [b]Department of Preventive, Restorative and Pediatric Dentistry, School of Dental Medicine, University of Bern, Bern, Switzerland

Abstract

During and after an erosive challenge, behavioral factors play a role in modifying the extent of erosive tooth wear. The manner that dietary acids are introduced into the mouth (gulping, sipping, use of a straw) will affect how long the teeth are in contact with the erosive challenge. The frequency and duration of exposure to an erosive agent is of paramount importance. Night-time exposure (e.g. baby bottle-feeding) to erosive agents may be particularly destructive because of the absence of salivary flow. Health-conscious individuals tend to ingest acidic drinks and juices more frequently and tend to have higher than average oral hygiene. While good oral hygiene is of proven value in the prevention of periodontal disease and dental caries, frequent toothbrushing with abrasive oral hygiene products may enhance erosive tooth wear. Unhealthy lifestyles such as consumption of designer drugs, alcopops and alcohol abuse are other important behavioral factors.

The clinical expression of dental erosion is highly variable with some individuals experiencing total destruction of their teeth and others maintaining most of their tooth structure throughout their lifetime [1]. While the evidence linking exposure of endogenous and exogenous acids to dental erosion is very strong, it is clear that that the clinical manifestation is modified by biological and behavioral factors. If this were not the case, then the prevalence of erosion would be much higher since many of us consume acid beverages and experience exposure to gastric acids at some time in our lives. Biological factors (covered in the chapter 7.1.2 by Hara et al., this vol, pp 88–99) likely account for some of the variability. However, differences in lifestyle and behavior are also important in the etiology of dental erosion [1]. Behavioral factors which can modify the extent of tooth wear include abusive or unusual consumption of

Table 1. Behavioral factors influencing erosive tooth wear

- Unusual eating and drinking habits
- Healthier life style: diets high in acidic fruits and vegetables
- Unhealthy life style: frequent consumption of alcopops and designer drugs
- Alcoholic disease
- Excessive consumption of acidic foods and drinks
- Night-time baby bottle feeding with acidic beverages
- Oral hygiene practices

foods and beverages, healthier lifestyles that may involve frequent consumption of acidic fruits and vegetables, frequent dieting with high consumption of citrus fruits and fruit juices as part of a weight-reducing plan, unhealthy lifestyles involving illegal designer drugs, overzealous oral hygiene practices with abrasive dentifrices, and excessive use of tooth bleaching/whitening products [1, 2]. Behavior can also be strongly influenced by socioeconomic status. Several studies have evaluated the relationship between socioeconomic status and dental erosion [3, 4], but there is a need for more definitive studies in this area. This chapter will focus on the dietary behavioral factors which influence the clinical expression of dental erosion (table 1).

Abusive or Unusual Consumption of Foods and Beverages

There is a wide range of foods and beverages that can contribute to erosive tooth wear [1]. The chemical and physical properties of acidic foods and beverages that contribute to their erosive potential have been covered in the chapter 7.1.1 by Lussi et al. (this vol, pp 77–87). Generally, the moderate consumption of even highly acidic foods and beverages does not necessarily lead to erosive tooth wear progression in individuals unless there are other modifying factors such as markedly decreased salivary gland function. Behaviors which increase the contact time of an acidic substance with teeth are likely to be the main driving force leading to erosion in many individuals.

There are many accounts of abusive or unusual behavior by individuals who frequently ingested acidic fruit juices or carbonated beverages, which have been linked to excessive dental erosion [5–9]. More recent studies have increasingly linked high consumption of carbonated drinks with increased risk of developing erosion [10–12]. Excessive consumption of acidic candies combined with a low salivary buffering capacity may aggravate erosive lesions [13, 14]. Excessive consumption of acidic fruits such as oranges has also been correlated with dental erosion [15].

Unusual eating and drinking methods, as well as swallowing habits which increase the direct contact time of acidic foods and beverages with the teeth, are obvious factors that will increase the risk of dental erosion. The manner that dietary acids are introduced into the mouth (gulping, sipping, use of a straw) will affect which teeth are in contact with the erosive challenge and possibly the clearance pattern [16, 17]. Holding drinks in the mouth before swallowing causes a marked pH drop at the tooth surface and increases the risk of erosion [18]. Several authors have suggested that using a straw is beneficial, since the straw directs drinks past the anterior teeth and towards the pharynx [17, 19, 20]. However, the placing of a straw labial to the anterior teeth can be very destructive [21]. The time of day of exposure to an erosive challenge is also important. Bedtime exposure to acid beverages poses a specific risk factor for children [22]. Exposure to erosive agents at night is particularly destructive because of the nocturnal absence of salivary flow.

Healthier Lifestyles

The pursuit of a healthier lifestyle, paradoxically, can lead to dental health problems in the form of dental erosion. The pursuit of 'healthier' lifestyles can involve regular exercise and what is considered healthy diets with more fruits and vegetables. The benefits of exercise are well proven; however, exercise increases the loss of body fluids and may lead to dehydration and decreased salivary flow. Satisfying an increased energy requirement and need for fluid intake with low-pH sugar-containing beverages during a time of decreased salivary flow may be doubly dangerous to the dentition. Frequent ingestion of acidic sports drinks, fruit juices and other carbonated and uncarbonated acidic beverages may therefore increase the risk of dental erosion for the athlete [23]. A recent review indicated that the evidence for an association between sports drinks and risk for dental erosion was not as strong as for other acidic beverages [24]. There may also be an overlap with an intrinsic etiologic factor. Vigorous exercise has been shown to increase the possibility of gastroesophageal reflux in some individuals [25].

Healthier diets include the consumption of more fruits and vegetables. A lactovegetarian diet, which includes the consumption of acidic foods, has been associated with a higher prevalence of dental erosion [26]. Individuals that live on a raw food diet have been shown to have significantly more dental erosion. Vegetarianism is also common in certain ethnic and religious groups [27]. Some herbal teas, particularly brands containing rose hip, lemon and mallow, were found to be very acidic (pH 2.6–3.9), with a relatively high buffering capacity and a low fluoride concentration [28]. Herbal teas, widely perceived as a healthy drink, may have an erosive potential exceeding that of orange juice [29]. Many iced tea products also have added lemon juice or citric acid and thus have the potential to cause dental erosion [30, 31].

Frequent dieting for health or vanity is another behavioral pattern that is common in many Western countries. A high consumption of citrus fruits and fruit juices may be part of weight reduction plans which can increase the risk for dental erosion. Also, fasting for health reasons may involve the frequent consumption of herbal teas. Angmar-Månsson and Oliveby [28] suggested that the combination of consuming acidic drinks and reduced salivary flow associated with fasting may increase the risk of dental erosion.

To further compound the problem, health conscious individuals also tend to have better than average oral hygiene. While good oral hygiene is of proven value in the prevention of periodontal disease and dental caries, frequent toothbrushing with abrasive oral hygiene products may render teeth more susceptible to dental erosion [1] (see chapter 3 by Addy et al., this vol, pp 17–31). Several studies have shown that the loss of tooth substance after exposure to citrus fruit juice is accelerated by toothbrushing [32]. The clinical implication of this is that toothbrushing surface immediately after ingestion of acidic foods or beverages may accelerate tooth loss (see chapter 12 by Lussi et al., this vol, pp 190–199).

Unhealthy Lifestyles

At the other end of the spectrum, an unhealthy lifestyle may also be associated with dental erosion. Alcoholics may be at particular risk for dental erosion and tooth wear. Robb and Smith [33] reported significantly more tooth wear in 37 alcoholic patients than in age- and sex-matched controls. Tooth wear was most pronounced in males and those with frequent alcohol consumption. Above all, the palatal surfaces of the upper anterior teeth showed erosive tooth wear which in most cases was connected to gastrointestinal symptoms and vomiting. Associations have also been found between dental erosions and the duration of alcoholic abuse and with symptoms and disease of the gastrointestinal tract [34]. In another study [35], prevalence of tooth erosion was 47.1% in alcohol abusers. Also of concern is the increased use of alcoholic soft drinks (alcopops) by adolescence children and young adults, which in addition to the potential of inducing vomiting are highly acidic [36, 37]. There is some evidence that cider is erosive [38, 39].

Dental erosion has also been associated with individuals that use illegal designer drugs. Duxbury [40] suggested that the use of 'ecstasy' (3,4-methylenedioxy-methamphetamine) may be a contributing factor to dental disease. The combination of ecstasy-induced dry mouth, dehydration from the vigorous physical activity, and the excessive consumption of low pH soft drinks may result in an increased likelihood of dental erosion and dental caries.

References

1   Zero DT: Etiology of dental erosion-extrinsic factors. Eur J Oral Sci 1996;104:162–177.
2   Zero DT, Lussi A: Etiology of enamel erosion – intrinsic and extrinsic factors. (chapter); in Addy M, Embery G, Edgar M, Orchardson R (eds): Tooth Wear and Sensitivity. London, Martin Dunitz, 2000, pp 121–139.
3   Millward A, Shaw L, Smith AJ, Rippin JW, Harrington E: The distribution and severity of tooth wear and the relationship between erosion and dietary constituents in a group of children. Int J Paediatr Dent 1994;4:152–157.
4   Milosevic A, Young PJ, Lennon MA: The prevalence of tooth wear in 14-year-old school children in Liverpool. Community Dent Health 1994;11:83–86.
5   High AS: An unusual pattern of dental erosion: a case report. Br Dent J 1977;143:403–404.
6   Mueninghoff LA, Johnson MH: Erosion: a case caused by unusual diet. J Am Diet Assoc 1982;104:51–52.
7   Mackie IC, Hobson P: Case reports: dental erosion associated with unusual drinking habits in childhood. J Paediatr Dent 1986;2:89–94.
8   Asher C, Read MJF: Early enamel erosion in children associated with excessive consumption of citric acid. Br Dent J 1987;162:384–387.
9   Harrison JL, Roder LB: Dental erosion caused by cola beverages. Gen Dent 1991;39:23–24.
10 Johansson AK, Lingström P, Birkhed D: Comparison of factors potentially related to the occurrence of dental erosion in high- and low-erosion groups. Eur J Oral Sci 2002;110:204–211.
11 Jensdottir T, Arnadottir IB, Thorsdottir I, Bardow A, Gudmundsson K, Theodors A, Holbrook WP: Relationship between dental erosion, soft drink consumption, and gastroesophageal reflux among Icelanders. Clin Oral Investing 2004;8:91–96.
12 Dugmore CR, Rock WP: A multifactorial analysis of factors associated with dental erosion. Br Dent J 2004;196:283–286.
13 Distler W, Bronner H, Hickel R, Petschelt A: Die Säurefreisetzung beim Verzehr von zuckerfreien Fruchtbonbons in der Mundhöhle in vivo. Dtsch Zahn Z 1993;48:492–494.
14 Lussi A, Portmann P, Burhop B: Erosion on abraded dental hard tissues by acid lozenges: an in situ study. Clin Oral Invest 1997;1:191–194.
15 Künzel W, Cruz MS, Fischer T: Dental erosion in Cuban children associated with excessive consumption of oranges. Eur J Oral Sci 2000;108:104–109.
16 Millward A, Shaw L, Harrington E, Smith AJ: Continuous monitoring of salivary flow rate and pH at the surface of the dentition following consumption of acidic beverages. Caries Res 1997;31: 44–49.
17 Edwards M, Ashwood RA, Littlewood SJ, Brocklebank LM, Fung DE: A videofluoroscopic comparison of straw and cup drinking: the potential influence on dental erosion. Br Dent J 1998;185:244–249.
18 Johansson AK, Lingström P, Imfeld T, Birkhed D: Influence of drinking method on tooth-surface pH in relation to dental erosion. Eur J Oral Sci 2004;112:484–489.
19 Grobler SR, Jenkins GN, Kotze D: The effects of the composition and method of drinking of soft drinks on plaque pH. Br Dent J 1985;158:293–296.
20 Imfeld T: Prevention of progression of dental erosion by professional and individual prophylactic measures. Eur J Oral Sci 1996;104:215–220.
21 Mackie IC, Blinkhorn AS: Unexplained losses of enamel on upper incisor teeth. Dent Update 1989;16:403–404.
22 Millward A, Shaw L, Smith A: Dental erosion in four-year-old children from differing socio-economic backgrounds. J Dent Child 1994;61:263–266.
23 Young WG: Diet and nutrition for oral health: advice for patients with tooth wear. Aust Dent Assoc News Bull 1995;July:8–10.

24 Coombes JS: Sports drinks and dental erosion. Am J Dent 2005;18:101–104.

25 Clark CS, Kraus BB, Sinclair J, Castell DO: Gastroesophageal reflux induced by exercise in healthy volunteers. JAMA 1989;261:3599–3601.

26 Ganss C, Schlechtriemen M, Klimek J: Dental erosions in subjects living on a raw food diet. Caries Res 1999;33:74–80.

27 Smith BNG, Knight JK: A comparison of pattern of tooth wear with aetiological factors. Br Dent J 1984;157:16–19.

28 Angmar-Månsson B, Oliveby A: Herbal tea – an erosion risk? pH, buffer capacity and fluoride concentration of herbal tea. Tandlakartidningen 1980;72:1315–1317.

29 Phelan J, Rees J: The erosive potential of some herbal teas. J Dent 2003;31:241–246.

30 Behrendt A, Oberste V, Wetzel WE: Fluoride concentration and pH of iced tea products. Caries Res 2002;36:405–410.

31 Willershausen B, Schulz-Dobrick B: In vitro study on dental erosion provoked by various beverages using electron probe microanalysis. Eur J Med Res 2004;9:432–438.

32 Davis WB, Winter PJ: The effect of abrasion on enamel and dentine after exposure to dietary acids. Br Dent J 1980;148:253–256.

33 Robb ND, Smith BG: Prevalence of pathological tooth wear in patients with chronic alcoholism. Br Dent J 1990;169:367–369.

34 Hede B: Determinants of oral health in a group of Danish alcoholics. Eur J Oral Sci 1996;104: 403–408.

35 Araujo MW, Dermen K, Connors G, Ciancio S: Oral and dental health among inpatients in treatment for alcohol use disorders: a pilot study. J Int Acad Periodontol 2004;6:125–130.

36 O'Sullivan EA, Curzon ME: Dental erosion associated with the use of 'alcopop': a case report. Br Dent J 1998;184:594–596.

37 Rees JS, Burford K, Loyn T: The erosive potential of the alcoholic lemonade Hooch. Eur J Prosthodont Restor Dent 1998;6:161–164.

38 Mathew T, Casamassimo PS, Hayes JR: Relationship between sports drinks and dental erosion in 304 university athletes in Columbus, Ohio, USA. Caries Res 2002;36:281–287.

39 Rees JS, Griffiths J: An in vitro assessment of the erosive potential of conventional and white ciders. Eur J Prosthodont Restor Dent 2002;10:167–171.

40 Duxbury AJ: Ecstasy: dental Implications. Br Dent J 1993;175:38.

Prof. Dr. Dominick Zero
Department of Preventive and Community
Dentistry, Indiana University
School of Dentistry
415 N. Lansing Street
Indianapolis, IN 46202-2876 (USA)

Lussi A (ed): Dental Erosion.
Monogr Oral Sci. Basel, Karger, 2006, vol 20, pp 106–111

....

Occupation and Sports

Adrian Lussi, Thomas Jaeggi

Department of Preventive, Restorative and Pediatric Dentistry,
School of Dental Medicine, University of Bern, Bern, Switzerland

Abstract

In rare cases the occupation – be it at work or during professional and strenuous sports activities – may give a clue to a patient's risk factors for dental erosion. However, no detrimental effects were described on a population level. Frequent contact to inorganic or organic acids at work could increase the occurrence and progression of erosion. In some studies, acid workers had significantly more teeth with erosive tooth wear than the controls. Clinical findings showed erosion mainly on upper anterior teeth and dentine hypersensitivity. Occupation groups at risk would mostly be found in the chemical industry, but also others like wine tasters may have dental erosion. A few case reports and studies have reported an association between sports activities and erosive tooth wear. The cause could be direct acid exposure or strenuous exercise, which may increase gastroesophageal reflux. Risk groups are swimmers exercising in water with low pH and athletes consuming frequently erosive sport drinks. It has to be kept in mind that sports drinks and occupation can be for some patients a cofactor in the development or in the increase of dental erosion. However, it is unlikely that one or two isolated factors will be responsible for this multifactorial condition.

Frequent contact to acids at the working place could increase the occurrence and/or the severity of dental erosion. When battery chargers were compared to automobile mechanics in Ibadan, Nigeria, 41% of the battery chargers' teeth had tooth wear whereas this number was 3% with mechanics [1]. A comparable finding was found in Jordan in the phosphate industry. The acid workers not only showed erosion but also complained in 80% of the cases about dentine hypersensitivity [2]. Acid fumes at work seem to be associated with tooth surface loss with no clinical significant differences between the inorganic and organic acids. Tuominen et al. [3–5] investigated the effect of inorganic and organic acid fumes on teeth. Among 169 workers who participated in one study, 88 were exposed to acid fumes and 81 were controls (not exposed to acid fumes). The prevalence of tooth surface loss was 63% (workers exposed to inorganic acid) and 50% (workers exposed to organic acid). The corresponding prevalence data for the controls were about 25%. The acid workers had significantly more teeth with erosive defects in the maxilla than the controls. Upper anterior teeth were more often attacked than posterior teeth. The purpose of another study [6] was to evaluate the prevalence and the severity of dental erosion and attrition in relation to exposure of airborne acids in the work environment. Measurements at a German battery factory showed that the workers were exposed to sulfuric acids (0.4–4.1 mg/cm^3). Erosion was found only in front teeth while attrition also occurred in posterior teeth. Due to the high level of crown restorations a rather moderate dose–effect relationship was observed. The authors concluded that severe erosion and attrition due to sulfuric acid mists should be recognized as an occupational disease.

Westegaard et al. [7] examined 425 individuals working at a pharmaceutical and biotechnological enterprise. Two hundred and two of these individuals were newly employed by the company and served as a control. Adjusted for potential confounders, there was no association between history of occupational exposure to proteolytic enzymes and prevalent facial or lingual erosion. With respect to prevalence of class V restorations, the association was significant. This study did not support the hypothesis that occupational exposure to airborne proteolytic enzymes is associated with dental erosions.

Wine has properties such as low pH, low content of P and Ca, which renders it to have an erosive potential (see chapter 7.1.1 by Lussi et al., this vol, pp 77–87). Professional wine tasting is very common all over the world. In some countries (e.g. Sweden, Finland) wine tasters are employed by the state to support their state-owned wine shops. Full-time Swedish wine tasters test on average 20–50 different wines, nearly 5 days a week. Wiktorsson et al. [8] investigated the prevalence and severity of tooth erosion in 19 qualified wine tasters in relation to number of years of wine tasting, salivary flow rate and buffer capacity. Salivary flow rate and buffer capacity of unstimulated and stimulated saliva were measured. Data on occupational background and dental and medical histories were collected. Fourteen subjects had tooth erosion mainly on the labio-cervical surfaces of maxillary incisors and canines. The severity of the erosion tended to increase with years of occupational exposure. Caries activity in all subjects was low. It was concluded that full-time wine tasting is an occupation associated with an increased risk for tooth erosion. Thereafter, the wine tasters employed at the state owned 'Systembolaget' got free dental hygiene prophylactic treatment as erosion was considered to be a work-related condition (pers. commun. to the authors). Several case reports pointed out the increased dentine hypersensitivity, manifest hard tissue loss and the need of early diagnosis and prevention [9–11].

Chronic alcoholic patients often show erosion. Although a certain direct impact of the alcohol cannot be ruled out one has to keep in mind that alcoholics often have regurgitation, which explains the clinical appearance (see chapter 7.1.3 by Zero et al., this vol, pp 100–105).

During sports activities dehydration occurs and rehydration and electrolyte replacement is accomplished by sports drinks that have an erosive potential comparable to acidic soft drinks (see chapter 7.1.1 by Lussi et al., this vol, pp 77–87). However, for most individuals engaged in physical activity, sports drinks have no performance benefit over water [12]. Probably, the greatest benefit of sports drinks to exercising individuals is that they generally increase voluntary fluid consumption [13]. This may be important as during heavy sporting activities only 50% of the rate of fluid loss is compensated [14]. Dentists should counsel athletes to control the effect of potentially erosive drinks [15].

A few case reports and studies have reported an association between sports activities and dental erosion. In a study with 25 swimmers and 20 cyclists, the latter showed significantly more tooth wear into dentine. However, no association between erosive tooth wear and sports drinks consumption was found [16]. Professional swimmers train several hours in the water, which should have proper pH regulation. The main disinfection techniques used are gas chlorination and sodium hypochlorite. In the Netherlands where the sodium hypochlorite method is used, only 0.14% of the tested pools were found in the year 2001 to have low pH values [17]. Another case report confirmed these findings [18]. In a review by Geurtsen [19], an increased prevalence of dental erosion among intensive swimmers due to low pH gas-chlorinated pool water was described. The recommended pH for swimming pools is between pH 7.2 and 8.0. Swimming activities in pH-adjusted pools do not harm the teeth [20]. However, erosion among competitive swimmers was found in 39% of swim team members who trained in a pool with a pH of 2.7 which is an H^+ concentration 100,000 times higher than that recommended for swimming pools [21].

In a patient complaining of severe dentine hypersensitivity, her case history revealed that she was an active diver over many years with 25 h/week training in chlorinated water and drank 1 l/day of an acidic soft drink sip-wise. Only later did she admit that she also had regurgitation which was an important factor explaining the clinical appearance of her teeth. Indeed, strenuous exercise may increase reflux [22]. Unstimulated saliva flow rate was high (1.2 ml/min) and the buffer capacity as measured with Dentobuff (Vivadent, Schaan, Liechtenstein) was 'medium'. Clinical examination showed severe erosive defects with involvement of dentine on all tooth surfaces (figs. 1–3). A one-bottle dentine adhesive was applied onto the hypersensitive teeth and the eroded parts of the teeth were filled with composite (for treatment procedures, see chapter 13 by Jaeggi et al., this vol, pp 200–214).

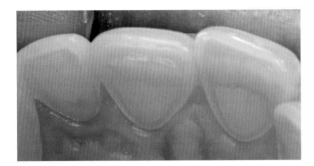

Fig. 1. Severe palatal erosive tooth wear with extensive dentinal exposure. Note the intact enamel along the gingival margin. Age of patient: 38 years, active diver in chlorinated water. Known risk factors: gastroesophageal reflux, acidic soft drinks sip-wise.

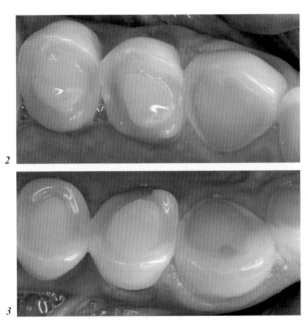

Fig. 2, 3. Severe oral and occlusal erosive tooth wear (same patient as fig. 1). Note the composite fillings rising above the level of the adjacent tooth surfaces.

A sample of athletes in the USA showed sports drinks usage in 92% of those and a total prevalence of erosion of 37%. Statistical analysis revealed no association between dental erosion and the use of sports drinks, quantity and frequency of consumption, years of usage and nonsport usage of sports drinks [23]. The prevalence found in this study was similar compared to that reported in a study with randomly selected persons using the same index [24]. This is a second indication that the consumption of these sports drinks did not increase the prevalence of erosion. A study in situ compared the erosive effect of a commercially available sports drink with that of mineral water over a 10-day period on 10 healthy volunteers. Erosion occurred with the sports drink, but to a variable degree between subjects [25]. In a recent in situ study, 19 healthy adults tested a commercially available sports drink, a calcium-enriched experimental sports drink, and natural mineral water during weekday exercise (75 min/day during 3 weeks). The total enamel surface loss was 4.2 μm for commercially available sports drinks, 0.14 μm for experimental sports drink and water [26]. Significant reduction of the erosive potential was found in two other studies where calcium or phosphopeptide-stabilized amorphous calcium phosphate was added [27, 28]. In both experiments, the pH of the test product was higher compared to the control.

Although no detrimental effects were described on a population level one has to keep in mind that sports drinks and occupation can be for some patients a cofactor in the development or in the increase of dental erosion when other factors are present. It is unlikely that one or two isolated factors (e.g. sports drink, dehydration) will be responsible for a multifactorial condition like erosion.

References

1   Arowojolu MO: Erosion of tooth enamel surfaces among battery chargers and automobile mechanics in Ibadan: a comparative study. Afr J Med Med Sci 2001;30:5–8.
2   Amin WM, Al-Omoush SA, Hattab FN: Oral health status of workers exposed to acid fumes in phosphate and battery industries in Jordan. Int Dent J 2001;51:169–174.
3   Tuominen M, Tuominen R, Ranta K, Ranta H: Association between acid fumes in the work environment and dental erosion. Scand J Work Environ Health 1989;15:335–338.
4   Tuominen M, Tuominen R, Fubusa F, Mgalula N: Tooth surface loss exposure to organic and inorganic acid fumes in workplace air. Community Dent Oral Epidemiol 1991;19:217–220.
5   Tuominen M, Tuominen R: Dental erosion and associated factors among factory workers exposed to inorganic acid fumes. Proc Finn Dent Soc 1991;87:359–364.
6   Petersen PE, Gormsen C: Oral conditions among German battery factory workers. Community Dent Oral Epidemiol 1991;19:104–106.
7   Westergaard J, Larsen IB, Holmen L, Larsen AI, Jorgensen B, Holmstrup P, Suadicani P, Gyntelberg F: Occupational exposure to airborne proteolytic enzymes and lifestyle risk factors for dental erosion-a cross-sectional study. Occup Med 2001;51:189–197.
8   Wiktorsson AM, Zimmerman M, Angmar-Mansson B: Erosive tooth wear: prevalence and severity in Swedish wine tasters. Eur J Oral Sci 1997;105:544–550.
9   Ferguson MM, Dunbar RJ, Smith JA, Wall JG: Enamel erosion related to wine making. Occup Med 1996;46:159–162.
10   Chaudhry SI, Harris JL, Challacombe SJ: Dental erosion in a wine merchant: an occupational hazard? Br Dent J 1997;182:226–228.
11   Gray A, Ferguson MM, Wall JG: Wine tasting and dental erosion: case report. Aust Dent J 1998;43:32–34.

12 Coombes JS, Hamilton KL: The effectiveness of commercially available sports drinks. Sports Med 2000;29:181–209.

13 Coombes JS: Sports drinks and dental erosion. Am J Dent 2005;18:101–104.

14 Pugh LG, Corbett JL, Johnson RH: Rectal temperatures, weight losses, and sweat rates in marathon running. J Appl Physiol 1967;23:347–352.

15 Sirimaharaj V, Brearley Messer L, Morgan MV: Acidic diet and dental erosion among athletes. Aust Dent J 2002;47:228–236.

16 Milosevic A, Kelly MJ, McLean AN: Sports supplement drinks and dental health in competitive swimmers and cyclists. Br Dent J 1997;182:303–308.

17 Lokin PA, Huysmans MC: Is Dutch swimming pool water erosive? Ned Tijdschr Tandheelkd 2004;111:14–16.

18 Scheper WA, van Nieuw Amerongen A, Eijkman MA: Oral conditions in swimmers. Ned Tijdschr Tandheelkd 2005;112:147–148.

19 Geurtsen W: Rapid general dental erosion by gas-chlorinated swimming pool water: review of the literature and case report. Am J Dent 2000;13:291–293.

20 Williams D, Croucher R, Marcenes W, O'Farrell M: The prevalence of dental erosion in the maxillary incisors of 14-year-old schoolchildren living in Tower Hamlets and Hackney, London, UK. Int Dent J 1999;49:211–216.

21 Centerwall BS, Armstrong CW, Funkhouser LS, Elzay RP: Erosion of dental enamel among competitive swimmers at a gas-chlorinated swimming pool. Am J Epidemiol 1986;123:641–647.

22 Clark CS, Kraus BB, Sinclair J, Castell DO: Gastroesophageal reflux induced by exercise in healthy volunteers. JAMA 1989;261:3599–3601.

23 Mathew T, Casamassimo PS, Hayes JR: Relationship between sports drinks and dental erosion in 304 university athletes in Columbus, Ohio, USA. Caries Res 2002;36:281–287.

24 Lussi A, Schaffner M, Hotz P, Suter P: Dental erosion in a population of Swiss adults. Community Dent Oral Epidemiol 1991;19:286–290.

25 Hooper SM, Hughes JA, Newcombe RG, Addy M, West NX: A methodology for testing the erosive potential of sports drinks. J Dent 2005;33:343–348.

26 Venables MC, Shaw L, Jeukendrup AE, Roedig-Penman A, Finke M, Newcombe RG, Parry J, Smith AJ: Erosive effect of a new sports drink on dental enamel during exercise. Med Sci Sports Exerc 2005;37:39–44.

27 Hooper SM, West NX, Sharif N, Smith S, North M, De'Ath J, Parker DM, Roedig-Penman A, Addy M: A comparison of enamel erosion by a new sports drink compared to two proprietary products: a controlled, crossover study in situ. J Dent 2004;32:541–545.

28 Ramalingam L, Messer LB, Reynolds EC: Adding case in phosphopeptide-amorphous calcium phosphate to sports drinks to eliminate in vitro erosion. Pediatr Dent 2005;27:61–67.

Prof. Dr. Adrian Lussi
Department of Preventive, Restorative and Pediatric Dentistry
School of Dental Medicine
University of Bern
Freiburgstrasse 7
CH–3010 Bern (Switzerland)

Chapter 7.3

Lussi A (ed): Dental Erosion.
Monogr Oral Sci. Basel, Karger, 2006, vol 20, pp 112–118

·······················

Oral Hygiene Products and Acidic Medicines

E. Hellwig[a], A. Lussi[b]

[a]Department of Operative Dentistry and Periodontology, University Clinic of Dentistry, Freiburg, Germany; [b]Department of Preventive, Restorative and Pediatric Dentistry, School of Dental Medicine, University of Bern, Bern, Switzerland

Abstract

Acidic or EDTA-containing oral hygiene products and acidic medicines have the potential to soften dental hard tissues. The low pH of oral care products increases the chemical stability of some fluoride compounds, favors the incorporation of fluoride ions in the lattice of hydroxyapatite and the precipitation of calcium fluoride on the tooth surface. This layer has some protective effect against an erosive attack. However, when the pH is too low or when no fluoride is present these protecting effects are replaced by direct softening of the tooth surface. Xerostomia or oral dryness can occur as a consequence of medication such as tranquilizers, anti-histamines, anti-emetics and anti-parkinsonian medicaments or of salivary gland dysfunction e.g. due to radiotherapy of the oral cavity and the head and neck region. Above all, these patients should be aware of the potential demineralization effects of oral hygiene products with low pH and high titratable acids. Acetyl salicylic acid taken regularly in the form of multiple chewable tablets or in the form of headache powder as well chewing hydrochloric acids tablets for treatment of stomach disorders can cause erosion. There is most probably no direct association between asthmatic drugs and erosion on the population level. Consumers, patients and health professionals should be aware of the potential of tooth damage not only by oral hygiene products and salivary substitutes but also by chewable and effervescent tablets. Additionally, it can be assumed that patients suffering from xerostomia should be aware of the potential effects of oral hygiene products with low pH and high titratable acids.

Erosive tooth wear is caused by different intrinsic and extrinsic acidic sources and may be modified by several factors (see chapter 1 by Lussi, this vol, pp 1–8). While much of the literature concerning erosive tooth wear deals with the influence of dietary, environmental and lifestyle factors, only scarce information is available about the contribution of medicaments and/or oral health products to erosive destruction of dental hard tissues. However, there are some reports in the literature describing acidic medicaments as etiological factor for the development of erosive lesions. Zero [1] in a review about the etiology of erosions mentioned iron tonics, liquid hydrochloric acid, vitamin C, aspirin, acidic oral hygiene products or products with calcium chelators, as well as acidic salivary substitutes and salivary flow stimulants as potential erosive products.

Oral Hygiene Products

Many oral care products such as toothpastes and fluoride-rinsing solutions exhibit a low pH. This, on the one hand, enhances the chemical stability of some fluoride compounds and, on the other, favors the incorporation of fluoride ions in the lattice of hydroxyapatite forming fluoridated hydroxyapatite (e.g. in white spot lesions). Furthermore, it favors the precipitation of calcium fluoride on the tooth surface. The formation of the latter on the tooth surface can act as a protection against acid attacks [2–4].

So far, the erosive potential of oral care products has been investigated in only a few studies: an EDTA-containing anti-calculus rinsing solution exhibited an erosive effect on enamel after a 2-h exposure time in vitro. This was explained by the calcium-chelating action of EDTA [5]. In another study, 11 commercially available rinsing solutions were examined for their acid content. The pH values found ranged between 3.4 and 8.3. Also, titration values ('buffer capacity') varied strongly among the solutions tested. Whether or not the solutions were likely to cause erosions was not investigated [6].

Pontefract et al. [7] performed an in situ and in vitro-study to measure enamel erosions by low pH mouthrinses. They used an acidified sodium chlorite mouthrinse (ASC, pH 3.02), an essential oil mouthrinse (Listerine®, pH 3.59), and a hexitidine mouthrinse (0.1%, pH 3.75). They compared the mouthrinses with orange juice and mineral water and found that all three rinses and orange juice led to a progressive enamel loss over time. ASC produced similar erosion as orange juice and significantly more erosion than the two proprietary rinses and water. The essential oil and the hexitidine mouthrinses produced similar erosions and significantly more mineral loss than water. This was substantiated in their in vitro study. Pretty et al. [8] could also show that Listerine caused erosion. The authors concluded that the patients should avoid using acidic mouth rinses as prebrushing rinses or following erosive challenges, e.g. vomiting.

In an in vitro model Meurman et al. [9] investigated the erosive effects of commercially available cotton swabs meant for hospital use and compared them to a saliva-stimulating chewing tablet. Disposable cotton swabs are often used for cleaning and moistening mouth and teeth in bedridden patients or otherwise disabled persons, who are not able to take care of their own daily oral hygiene. The authors could demonstrate that disposable cotton swabs with a low pH and a high acid content can cause tooth erosion. Repeated use of such swabs may therefore be detrimental to the teeth. Since bedridden and medically compromised patients often suffer from reduced saliva flow, the erosive effects may be enhanced in these cases. Consequently, those products should be avoided and less erosive products should be used as special mouth cleaning aids.

Lussi and Jaeggi [10] investigated the erosive potential of various oral care products and compared the results with those of various foodstuffs and beverages. In this in vitro study, they could show that among the dental hygiene products only the fluoride-free Weleda toothpaste led to a significant reduction of hardness. They suggested that Weleda softened the tooth surface due to its content of citric acid/citrate and the absence of fluoride in combination with its low pH of 3.7. Although some of the tested products (Elmex gelée®, Meridol dentifrice®, Meridol mouthrinse®) had a pH below 5, none of them showed surface softening. Attin et al. [2] could also demonstrate that the application of a fluoride containing gel with a pH of 4.75 (Elmex gelée) increased the abrasion resistance of eroded enamel. Lussi and Jaeggi [10] suggested that after topical application of acidic oral hygiene products with a high fluoride content some mineral is dissolved from the enamel surface, thereby increasing the local pH and leading to reprecipitation of fluoridated hydroxyapatite. Moreover, the buffer capacity of saliva and the organic pellicle led to an additional protective effect. It seems that highly concentrated slightly acidic fluoride applications are able to increase abrasion resistance and decrease the development of erosions of enamel and dentin. Wiegand et al. [11] showed that toothbrush abrasion of eroded dentin may be influenced by the fluoride content, by the RDA value and particularly by the buffer capacity of the applied dentifrice or gel.

A different problem arises in patients suffering from xerostomia or oral dryness as a consequence of medication or of salivary gland dysfunction. These individuals sip liquids frequently to eliminate the discomfort associated with reduced saliva. Samarawickrama [12] stated that a properly balanced saliva substitute may become necessary to manage xerostomia when no means of stimulating the saliva are effective. This product should have a neutral pH and contain electrolytes to make the composition similar to natural saliva. Xerostomia and oral dryness is a side effect of a wide variety of drugs such as anti-depressants, anti-hypertension, anti-psychotics and anti-histamines [13, 14]. Further, it is one of the most common complaints experienced by patients who underwent radiotherapy of the oral cavity and the head and neck region or who suffer from Sjogren's syndrome. Since the protective effects of saliva, e.g. buffer capacity and oral clearance is limited in those patients, salivary substitutes or oral hygiene products (mouthrinses, fluoride gels, etc.) with a low pH and a high amount of titratable acid lead to a progressive demineralization of dental hard tissues [15, 16]. Kielbassa et al. [17] found that Biotene® with a pH of 4.15 and Glandosane® with a pH of 4.08 led to mineral loss in enamel and in dentine. They concluded that fluoridated saliva substitutes containing mucins, phosphate and calcium are suitable for the relief of the symptoms of extensive xerostomia.

Acidic Medicines

If a medicine low in pH and high in titratable acidity is used frequently and/or over a long period of time, it has the potential to produce erosive lesions in teeth. Additionally, some medicines can contribute to increase the danger of erosion when reducing the salivary flow rate and/or buffer capacity of the saliva, e.g. tranquilizers, anti-histamines, anti-emetics and anti-parkinsonian medicaments [13, 14]. Nunn et al. [18] assessed eight liquid oral medicines and two effervescent preparations routinely prescribed for long-term use by pediatric renal patients with respect to pH values and titratable acid. They found that some of the medicines and particularly the two effervescent tablets showed low pH-values. Titratable acidity for hydralazine hydrochloride solution and Phosphate Sandoz® and Sandoz K® effervescent tablets were critical compared to the other medicaments. They concluded that health professionals need to be aware of the erosive potential of liquid oral medicines and recommend the use of tablets whenever that option exists.

The high popularity to use supplemental vitamin C (L-ascorbic acid), prescribed either professionally or self-prescribed, has increased during the last years. There are different preparations on the market, e.g. chewing tablets, syrup, effervescent vitamin C tablets. Giunta [19] concluded from a case report and from an in vitro test that chewable vitamin C tablets can cause a pH less than 2.0 in the oral cavity and that the pH of saliva can drop while chewing vitamin C tablets. Although the pH level varies from manufacturer to manufacturer, the level of acidity in vitamin C preparations is always high. Since tablets are hard, large and chewable, the time and the area of contact with the teeth may be high. Passon and Jones [20] reported a case of a 58-year-old man who took a 500-mg chewable vitamin C tablet daily over a period of 1 year. This man suffered from severe erosion of the upper and lower left canines and premolars where he held the tablets while he let them slowly dissolve. Consumers should be aware of the potential of tooth damage by chewable tablets and a physician should recommend vitamin C in a form which is safe. This is in accordance with the findings of Meurman and Murtomaa [21] who stated that for individuals with normal salivary flow the consumption of vitamin C preparations should not have erosive effects, unless the preparations are left in direct contact with the teeth. Results from clinical surveys suggest a strong positive correlation between the consumption of vitamin C supplements and the prevalence of erosions [22–24].

Erosion can also result from chronic use of chewable aspirin tablets or headache powder. McCracken and O'Neal [25] reported a 30-year-old female patient with a 3-year-history of headache powder use at six doses a day, each dose containing 520 mg aspirin. She placed the undissolved powder sublingually to increase the rate of absorption. Oral examination revealed severe erosion on the occlusal surfaces of the mandibular molars and premolars. Rogalla et al. [26] assessed the erosive action of unbuffered and buffered acetyl salicylic acid on tooth hard tissues in vitro. Scanning electron microscopy analysis of the enamel and dentine surfaces showed marked differences in the degree of erosion depending on the duration of exposure and the concentration of acetyl salicylic acid. They suggested that remnants of chewable tablets can stick in deep fissures, thereby exerting a long-lasting erosive effect. Their results are supported by a report published by Grace et al. [27], who showed that tooth erosion can be caused by chewable aspirin tablets. Particular patients with juvenile rheumatic arthritis who took aspirin in form of multiple chewable tablets per day experienced erosion on the occlusal surface, compared to children who swallowed the tablets and had no erosions [28].

Conflicting results concerning the association between asthma and tooth erosion were published [29–31]. Dugmore and Rock [31] in a representative random sample of adolescents in the UK found no association between asthma and tooth erosion. They also reported that 88% of drugs prescribed for asthma had a pH above 5.5. However, some drugs inhaled to combat asthma have a pH low enough to cause erosion, particularly when they come in frequent and/or sustained contact with teeth. When asthma medication is taken from an inhaler, the lips form a seal around the nozzle of the inhaler covering and protecting the labial surfaces of the incisors and canine teeth. Consequently, it is unlikely that any acidic medicaments would spread to the labial surfaces of the teeth subsequent to inhalation [31]. The authors listed a number of factors leading to erosion in asthmatic patients. The acidic nature of the medication is able to act directly on the teeth. Prolonged use of β_2-adrenoreceptor stimulants such as salbutamol, salmeterol or terbutaline leads to decreased salivary flow, thus reducing the modifying and protective effects of saliva. Drugs used as bronchodilatators act to relax smooth muscle. This may effect the esophageal sphincter in addition to the bronchus and thereby potentiate the gastroesophageal reflux, which is a recognized etiological factor in tooth erosion. The patients might increase their consumption of acidic drinks in an attempt to compensate for reduced saliva flow, increased dry mouth and the taste of drugs. The authors concluded that it is difficult to support an association between such drugs and the erosion on the population level. They also stated that most asthma inhalation medicaments are not acidic and pose no threat to the dentition. There seems to be no clear evidence of an association between decreased salivary flow rate due to asthma medication and tooth erosion. The proportion of drugs used that may promote gastro-esophageal reflux is low and unlikely to have a significant influence on tooth erosion prevalence. And they could not approve the thesis that asthmatic children consume more potentially erosive drinks than non-asthmatics. Sivasithamparam et al. [32] in a case control study from South East Queensland supported their conclusions. They found also no differences between asthmatics and other patients concerning citrus fruit and acidic soft drink consumption. They also found that gastro-esophageal reflux does not appear to contribute in a side-specific manner to erosion in asthmatics.

HCl tablets are used in order to treat stomach disorders and have also been cited as a cause of enamel erosion. Maron [33] described the case of severe enamel erosion caused after chewing hydrochloric acid tablets over a 5-year period. He concluded that dentists must be aware that highly erosive acids are obtainable without prescription, and that the misuse of acidic medicine might be responsible for severe erosive destruction of tooth hard tissues. In the reported case, a woman chewed the hydrochloric acid tablets rather than swallowing them.

References

1 Zero DT: Etiology of dental erosion: extrinsic factors. Eur J Oral Sci 1996;104:162–177.
2 Attin T, Deifuss H, Hellwig E: Influence of acidified fluoride gel on abrasion resistance of eroded enamel. Caries Res 1999;33:135–139.
3 Ganss C, Klimek J, Schäfer U, Spall T: Effectiveness of two fluoridation measures on erosion progression in human enamel and dentine in vitro. Caries Res 2001;35:325–330.
4 Lussi A, Jaeggi T, Schaffner M: Prevention and minimally invasive treatment of erosions. Oral Health Prev Dent 2004;2:321–325.
5 Rytömaa I, Meurman JH, Franssila S, Torkko H: Oral hygiene products may cause dental erosion. Proc Finn Dent Soc 1989;85:161–166.
6 Bhatti SA, Walsh TF, Douglas CW: Ethanol and pH levels of proprietary mouthrinses. Community Dent Health 1994;11:71–74.
7 Pontefract H, Hughes J, Kemp K, et al: The erosive effects of some mouthrinses on enamel: a study in situ. J Clin Periodontol 2001;28:319–324.
8 Pretty IA, Edgar WM, Higham SM: The erosive potential of commercially available mouthrinses on enamel as measured by quantitative light-induced fluorescence (QLF). J Dent 2003;31:313–319.
9 Meurman JH, Sorvari R, Pelttari A, Rytömaa I, Franssila S, Kroon L: Hospital mouth-cleaning aids may cause dental erosion. Spec Care Dentist 1996;16:247–250.
10 Lussi A, Jaeggi T: The erosive potential of various oral care products compared to foodstuffs and beverages. Schweiz Monatsschr Zahnmed 2001;111:274–281.
11 Wiegand A, Wolmershauser S, Hellwig E, Attin T: Influence of buffering effects of dentifrices and fluoride gels on abrasion on eroded dentine. Arch Oral Biol 2004;49:259–265.
12 Samarawickrama DY: Saliva substitutes: how effective and safe are they? Oral Dis 2002;8:177–179.

13   Atkinson JC, Wu AJ: Salivary gland dysfunction: causes, symptoms, treatment. Am Dent Assoc 1994;125:409–416.

14   Cassolato SF, Turnbull RS: Xerostomia: clinical aspects and treatment. Gerodontology 2003;20: 64–77.

15   Meyer-Lueckel H, Kielbassa AM: Use of saliva substitutes in patients with xerostomia. Schweiz Monatsschr Zahnmed 2002;112:1037–1058.

16   Kielbassa AM, Shohadai SP: Die Auswirkungen von Speichelersatzmitteln auf die Läsionstiefe von demineralisiertem Schmelz. Dtsch Zahnärzt Z 1999;54:757–763.

17   Kielbassa AM, Shohadai SP, Schulte-Monting J: Effect of saliva substitutes on mineral content of demineralized and sound dental enamel. Support Care Cancer 2001;9:40–47.

18   Nunn JH, Ng SK, Sharkey I, Coulthard M: The dental implications of chronic use of acidic medicines in medically compromised children. Pharm World Sci 2001;23:118–119.

19   Giunta JL: Dental erosion resulting from chewable vitamin C tablets. J Am Dent Assoc 1983;107:253–256.

20   Passon JC, Jones GK: Atypical dental erosion: a case report. Gerodontics 1986;2:77–79.

21   Meurman JH, Murtomaa H: Effect of effervescent vitamin C preparations on bovine teeth and on some clinical and salivary parameters in man. Scand J Dent Res 1986;94:491–499.

22   O'Sullivan EA, Curzon ME: A comparison of acidic dietary factors in children with and without dental erosion. ASDC J Dent Child 2000;67:186–192.

23   Al-Malik MI, Holt RD, Bedi R: The relationship between erosion, caries and rampant caries and dietary habits in preschool children in Saudi Arabia. Int J Paediatr Dent 2001;11:430–439.

24   Al-Dlaigan YH, Shaw L, Smith A: Dental erosion in a group of British 14-year-old school children. II. Influence of dietary intake. Br Dent J 2001;190:258–261.

25   McCracken M, O'Neal SJ: Dental erosion and aspirin headache powders: a clinical report. J Prosthodont 2000;9:95–98.

26   Rogalla K, Finger W, Hannig M: Influence of buffered and unbuffered acetylsalicylic acid on dental enamel and dentine in human teeth: an in vitro pilot study. Methods Find Exp Clin Pharmacol 1992;14:339–346.

27   Grace EG, Sarlani E, Kaplan S: Tooth erosion caused by chewing aspirin. J Am Dent Assoc 2004;135:911–914.

28   Sullivan RE, Kramer WS: Introgenic erosion of teeth. J Dent Child 1983;56:92–196.

29   Al-Dlaigan YH, Shaw L, Smith AJ: Is there a relationship between asthma and dental erosion? A case control study. Int J Paediatr Dent 2002;12:189–200.

30   Shaw L, al-Dlaigan YH, Smith A: Childhood asthma and dental erosion. ASDC J Dent Child 2000;67:102–106.

31   Dugmore CR, Rock WP: Asthma and tooth erosion: is there an association? Int J Paediatr Dent 2003;13:417–424.

32   Sivasithamparam K, Young WG, Jirattanasopa V, Priest J, Khan F, Harbrow D, Daley TJ, Sullivan RE, Kramer WS: Dental erosion in asthma: a case-control study from south east Queensland. Aust Dent J 2002;47:298–303.

33   Maron FS: Enamel erosion resulting from hydrochloric acid tablets. J Am Dent Assoc 1996;127: 781–784.

Prof. Dr. Elmar Hellwig
Department of Operative Dentistry and Periodontology
University Clinic of Dentistry, Freiburg
Hugstetter Strasse 55
DE–79106 Freiburg (Germany)

Lussi A (ed): Dental Erosion.
Monogr Oral Sci. Basel, Karger, 2006, vol 20, pp 119–139

....

Intrinsic Causes of Erosion

David Bartlett

Department of Prosthodontics, GKT Dental Institute, London, UK

Abstract

Gastric juice entering the mouth causes dental erosion. Common causes for the migration of gastric juice through the lower and upper oesophageal sphincters are reflux disease, eating disorders, chronic alcoholism and pregnancy. Gastro-oesophageal reflux is a common condition affecting up to 65% of the western population at some point in their lifetime. A typical clinical sign of acidic gastric juice entering the mouth is palatal dental erosion. As the condition becomes more chronic it becomes more widespread. There have been relatively few randomised studies investigating the aetiology of acids causing erosion. Of the few that have reported their findings, it appears that gastric acids are equally likely to induce moderate-to-severe erosion as in dietary acids. This literature review reports the conditions associated with the movement of gastric juice and dental erosion using medical and dental sources.

Hydrochloric acid produced by the parietal cells in the stomach causes intrinsic dental erosion. The acid reaches the mouth either through vomiting or by regurgitation. Vomiting disorders such as anorexia and bulimia nervosa have long been recognised as a factor in the development of dental erosion. More recently, regurgitation which is defined as involuntary movement of the gastric contents from the stomach into the mouth has also been acknowledged as a common cause of severe dental erosion. The palatal surfaces of the upper anterior teeth appear to be most commonly affected by the acid once it reaches the mouth. Early erosion appears as thinning of the enamel but as the condition persists dentine is eventually exposed and ultimately in severe cases the pulp is compromised. As the erosion continues, the destruction of enamel and dentine becomes more widespread and may not be limited to the palatal surfaces of the anterior teeth. The consequences of intrinsic erosion are often severe and require extensive restorative management to replace the lost tooth tissue.

There are a number of conditions associated with the movement of the gastric acid from the stomach to the mouth. An underlying common feature of most is gastro-oesophageal reflux (GOR). This is the term used to describe the retrograde movement of the stomach acid past the lower oesophageal sphincter. The condition is associated with other known causes of intrinsic erosion including rumination, chronic alcoholism, and eating disorders. Unlike dietary acids, the pH and titratability of gastric juice is significantly greater and so the level of destruction is normally more severe [1].

The most common presenting dental sign of gastric acid is the development of tooth wear on the palatal surfaces of the upper incisor teeth. In some cases, it is possible to identify the cause of the wear and associate it with gastric acid, particularly with eating disorders, but for most the cause is less certain. In these circumstances, a thorough and comprehensive clinical examination is needed to assess the most likely cause of the wear [2]. However, even with some it is difficult to make an accurate diagnosis and be certain of the aetiology of the wear [3].

The association of gastric causes to the development of palatal tooth wear has been investigated by a number of researchers. One study investigated a randomly selected group of Swiss adults and diagnosed the cause of tooth wear. In this population, although severe palatal erosion was rare, multiple regression analysis showed that vomiting was associated with its development [4]. Other studies have also investigated groups of patients presenting with palatal erosion and found associations with gastric causes [3, 5]. The concept that palatal erosion is associated with gastric acid has also been supported by Scandinavian researchers in a number of studies [6, 7]. The association with GOR and dental erosion has been investigated by researchers in the UK [8, 9], USA [10–12] and Scandinavia [13].

The acidity of gastric acid regurgitated into the mouth has the potential to cause severe destruction of teeth [1]. Although dietary acids have also been associated with dental erosion the wear by gastric causes is often severe and widespread. Early erosion is seen with loss of enamel from the palatal surfaces of the upper incisors but as the erosion progresses, the palatal cusps and surfaces of the premolars and molars also become involved. Finally, more generalised erosion on the occlusal surfaces of molars and the facial surfaces of all teeth produces severe tooth wear. This in extreme circumstances can result in the total obliteration of the crowns of teeth by gastric acids. Under these circumstances, the treatment which may be required to restore the worn dentition is both expensive and clinically challenging (see chapter 13 by Jaeggi et al., this vol, pp 200–214); [14, 15].

Gastro-Oesophageal Reflux

Anatomy and Physiology of the Oesophagus
The human oesophagus is a hollow muscular tube about 25 cm long bounded by a muscular sphincter at each end. The lower oesophageal sphincters (LOS) and

upper oesophageal sphincters (UOS) are physical barriers to the retrograde movement of the gastric contents to the mouth and pulmonary system. The upper part of the oesophagus, including the UOS, is composed of striated muscle. The LOS is not an anatomical but a physiological sphincter and involves the diaphragm and muscle folds. At the gastro-oesophageal junction, there is an abrupt change from squamous to simple columnar epithelial cells with gastric glands and pits but the precise location of the squamocolumnar junction in relation to the LOS is variable [16]. This junction is an important site as pre-malignant changes to the epithelium called Barrett's oesophagitis have been associated with reflux disease [17].

The main function of the oesophagus is to control the passage of solids and fluids from the mouth to the stomach in a co-ordinated manner, clearing regurgitated material and preventing GOR. In normal swallowing, the pharynx pumps and propels a bolus from the oropharynx, across a relaxed UOS, and into the oesophagus. Following that, oesophageal peristalsis drives the bolus into the stomach through a relaxed LOS [18]. In healthy subjects, primary peristalsis is a series of co-ordinated propulsive contractions passing down the oesophagus at a speed of 2–5 cm/s to reach the stomach [19].

The main role of the LOS is to prevent the stomach contents from passing into the oesophagus. The LOS is about 2.5–3.5 cm long and is located in the abdomen and the chest. The LOS is not a tight sphincter and movement of the gastric contents into the distal oesophagus can occur. Transient movement of the gastric contents commonly occurs, often following meals, and is usually limited to the distal oesophagus. Any retrograde contents are normally cleared by swallowing or peristalsis [20]. Abnormalities of the muscular function of the oesophagus are termed motility disorders. The symptoms associated with GOR include heartburn, regurgitation, dysphagia and chest pain [21, 22]. The most common reasons for the symptoms are failure of the LOS to relax with swallowing or the loss of peristaltic activity in the oesophageal body [23].

The major role of the UOS is to protect the airway. Retrograde movement of reflux from the stomach is prevented from reaching the pharynx by the UOS. The sphincter is approximately 2–4 cm in length [24]. The surrounding anatomical structures form the UOS into an elongated or slit-like cross-sectional shape. This shape helps to limit any retrograde movement. Unlike the LOS, the UOS is composed of skeletal muscle and has a higher tonic pressure and so is more efficient at preventing regurgitation. In patients with regurgitation, there may be a low basal pressure of the UOS or transient inappropriate relaxations, in a similar manner as the LOS.

Gastro-Oesophageal Reflux Disease

The manifestations of gastro-oesophageal reflux disease (GORD) typically relate to the oesophagus (table 1). The commonest oesophageal symptoms are

Table 1. Manifestations of gastro-oesophageal reflux disease

Oesophageal symptoms of reflux	
Heartburn	– radiates along the oesophagus[a]
Epigastric pain	– centralised over the stomach
Regurgitation	– stomach contents passing into the mouth[a]
Dysphagia	– difficulty in swallowing
Extra-oesophageal symptoms of reflux	
Retrosternal pain	– non-cardiac pain
Asthma	– regurgitation into pulmonary system
Laryngeal	– chronic cough and sore throat
Hoarseness	– alteration of voice[a]
Globus	– feeling of something stuck in the throat

[a]Associated with dental erosion [8–10, 25].

heartburn, regurgitation, dysphagia and chest pain [25]. The least frequent symptom of GORD is dysphagia, and is often only reported in patients with long-standing disease [26]. Dysphagia is the result of oesophagitis, dysmotility and stricture formation closing the oesophageal lumen and so resisting the passage of food into the stomach. Heartburn is a substernal burning radiating pain along the length of the oesophagus often passing to the throat. Epigastric pain is a localised pain, which may radiate from the epigastrium (overlying the xiphisternum). Retrosternal or non-cardiac chest pain is also a common symptom and can be confused with cardiac disease [25]. Regurgitation is the reflux of gastric juice through the UOS and into the oral cavity.

Heartburn has been recognised as a classic symptom of GORD [27]. Nebel et al. [28] in a study of hospitalised subjects, non-hospitalised subjects and controls reported that 7% of normal individuals, 14% of hospitalised patients and 15% of outpatients complained of daily heartburn. A survey in the UK showed that nearly half of them complained of having heartburn at least once a month. It also revealed that 29% take medication at least once a month [29]. Despite most symptoms of GOR involving the oesophagus there are other extra-oesophageal symptoms which have dental implications.

Regurgitation

Regurgitation can be defined as 'the sudden, effortless return of gastric or oesophageal contents into the pharynx and implies UOS relaxation or insufficiency'. Regurgitation should be distinguished from vomiting which is the propulsion of the stomach contents, co-ordinated by the vomiting centre in the brain [30]. Once past the UOS, the regurgitated material can either enter the oral cavity or be aspirated by the pulmonary system. The UOS therefore has an important role in the prevention of high reflux.

Cardiac

Severe chest pain is a distressing and worrying symptom for patients and can present clinicians with a difficult differential diagnosis with heart disease. GOR can present as chest pain and is a common cause of non-cardiac chest pain or NCCP [8, 9, 31].

Chronic Cough

Chronic coughs linked to GORD can be the sole presentation of GORD [32]. Micro-aspiration of refluxate has been demonstrated to cause symptoms after acid enters the pulmonary system [32–35].

GORD-Related Asthma

Asthma has long been recognised as a debilitating complication of GORD. The complex pathology of asthma seems to overlap with GORD-related asthma [36–38].

Laryngeal

A variety of abnormalities has been linked to laryngopharyngeal reflux. Examples include oedema with erythema, laryngeal stenosis [39, 40], and vocal cord ulcers [25, 41]. The presence of refluxed gastric contents above the UOS is believed to cause the inflammation but this link is being increasingly questioned. This partly reflects the relatively rare occurrence of the finding.

Chronic Hoarseness

As distinct to chronic cough, some patients present with chronic hoarseness with no discernible cause. It is uncertain whether vocal cord irritation occurs by the direct action of acid or by chronic throat clearing and coughing resulting from oesophageal acid stimulating a vagally mediated reflex.

Globus

The sensation of a persistent painless lump or ball in the throat on swallowing without dysphagia (difficulty in swallowing) is termed globus and is derived from the Greek for ball. The literature suggests that there may be an association between globus and GORD [42].

Implications of Symptoms of Reflux and Dental Erosion

Although heartburn is the most common symptom of reflux disease, it does not correlate well to the development of dental erosion. There have been a couple of studies investigating the reporting of symptoms from patients and the presence of dental erosion particularly in Scandinavia [6, 13]. Both these studies investigated patients presenting with symptoms of reflux and then assessed the prevalence of erosion. A clear correlation between the presence of the reported symptoms and the existence of dental erosion was not observed. Part of the problem is the difficulty concerning the value of the reported symptoms of reflux in these subjects. Silent reflux is an increasingly recognised phenomena [43]. In one dental study, up to 25% of subjects presenting with dental erosion were observed to have pathological levels of reflux despite not having any symptoms [8].

Another study investigated patients attending a general hospital after referral for reflux-related symptoms. The severity of tooth wear was assessed using a modified Smith and Knight Index and the results were compared to a control group [9]. Although, no correlation was observed between heartburn and the presence of tooth wear there were some weak relationships between extra-oesophageal symptoms, particularly hoarseness, and the severity of the dental erosion. Whilst this study could not be considered definitive, it suggests that reflux passing through both lower and upper sphincters has the potential to cause dental erosion. From a dental management perspective, it is useful to record any symptoms of reflux particularly those associated with the UOS as it might indicate an underlying disease process and imply that gastric reflux is the cause of the dental erosion.

Mechanisms of Reflux

In health, the pH of the oesophagus varies between 5 and 7. GOR is defined internationally by gastroenterologists as episodes during which the pH in the oesophagus falls below 4 (table 2). In healthy subjects, brief episodes of physiological reflux occurs which are effectively cleared by oesophageal peristalsis and this occurs mainly after food intake (postprandial periods). In most healthy individuals, dietary excess and alcohol consumption usually late at night can cause some discomfort from reflux and is normally termed 'indigestion'. For patients with GORD the symptoms are more exaggerated and prolonged. A useful term is that the symptoms interfere with the quality of life. For these patients, the pH within the oesophagus drops below 4 for long periods of time. Gastro-enterologists use pH testing to quantify the reflux periods, assess the acidity of the pH and determine correlations between reflux and symptoms. Generally, manometry is performed simultaneously to assess motility and transient relaxations.

Table 2. Common factors related to reflux

Mechanisms involved with reflux
Reduced lower oesophageal sphincter pressure and oesophageal motility [52]

Factors precipitating reflux
Diet – onions, fatty foods, chocolate, peppermint, spicy foods and pickles [31]
Alcohol – reduces LOS tone, delays gastric emptying and increasing GOR [44].
  In addition it is also an irritant of the oesophageal mucosa
Posture – bending or lying down increases GOR [31, 86]
Exercise – heartburn and nausea can occur as a result of strenuous exercise

These symptoms, however, although unpleasant are transient and do not have any
  long-lasting effect [45]

Some lifestyle and dietary factors are known to provoke reflux. For many
people who have infrequent symptoms dietary excess can produce symptoms
which are time limited and do not interfere with the subject's quality of life.
But for those with GORD the symptoms are prolonged and require little
provocation.

Some of these factors are listed below:

Diet
A number of common dietary components have been associated with GOR
such as onions, fatty foods, chocolate, peppermint, spicy food, pickles, toma-
toes and coffee [31].

Alcohol
Alcohol is acknowledged as reducing the LOS tone and delaying gastric
emptying hence increasing the likelihood of GOR [44]. In addition, it is also an
irritant of the oesophageal mucosa.

Posture
Body position can influence GOR due to the prone position during sleep
impairing the clearance of acid, whereas a vertical position aids acid clearance
simply due to the force of gravity.

Exercise
Symptoms of GORD in particular heartburn and nausea can occur as a
result of strenuous exercise. These symptoms, although unpleasant, are transient and do not have any long-lasting effect [45].

Obesity

Increase in body weight is another factor in predisposing to GORD [46]. The increase in size results in raised intra-gastric pressure increasing the potential for reflux to occur.

The Implications of Diet and Dental Erosion

Whilst dietary control and avoidance is a recognised management with extrinsic erosion it is less so with conditions related to reflux disease. In symptomatic patients, it is common to find that they avoid any foods likely to provoke reflux. Subjects will readily admit to avoiding spicy or acidic foods because consuming them is painful. Therefore, someone who is under care by a gastroenterologist may already be avoiding many of the foods listed above. However, if the patients are not aware of the reflux problems, they may not be avoiding these foods and reflux might be increased.

Diagnosis of GORD

Persistent and prolonged heartburn and regurgitation are the most common and typical symptoms of GORD and their presence is often a good indication of the presence of GORD. However, even in the absence of these symptoms GORD cannot be excluded. It is a cyclical condition often being tolerated for many years before seeking specialist medical care. Many patients, particularly when the condition first manifests, self-medicate and do not seek specialist advice. However, if the condition becomes more chronic and uncomfortable they tend to seek medical intervention. Self-medication can involve purchasing over-the-counter anti-reflux medication without any special tests or medical intervention. In more persistent cases further investigation is warranted. Once specialist opinion has been sought, the most commonly used techniques used to investigate GORD are 24-h ambulatory pH monitoring and endoscopy.

Ambulatory pH monitoring, normally over 24 h, has become the gold standard for investigating reflux disease. Electrodes are used to record changes in pH within the oesophagus and detect acid reflux [20]. The electrodes are attached to narrow catheters and passed via the nose to a position 5 cm above the LOS. The data recorded by the pH electrodes are stored digitally and analysed using internationally recognised criteria. The patients normally have the test over 24 h and are allowed home to follow a near normal day. The ambulatory test attempts to replicate normality and provide the clinician with a quantitative assessment of the reflux disease.

Endoscopy on the other hand allows the visual examination of the oesophagus. It is undertaken to directly examine the presence of diaphragmatic herniation, inflammation or ulceration around the distal oesophagus using an endoscope. A positive finding implies that reflux is occurring although it remains a subjective opinion. The presence or absence of inflammation does not necessarily imply that reflux is occurring. The specificity and sensitivity of the 24-h pH test is around 80% whereas for endoscopy it is much less [47]. Endoscopy also does not provide any information about the efficiency of peristalsis or quantify oesophageal motility with any certainty.

Management and Treatment of GORD
There are three main methods of management of GORD:
- Conservative therapy
- Medication
- Surgery

Conservative therapies such as increasing the number of pillows, avoiding reflux provoking foods and meals before bed time, decreased alcohol consumption, cessation of smoking, reducing weight and reducing stress are all recognised anti-reflux strategies.

Over the last 20 years, medical and surgical treatment of GORD has been revolutionised firstly by H_2 receptor antagonists and secondly by proton pump inhibitors. These act by inhibiting the proton pump in the parietal cell, causing powerful and sustained inhibition of gastric secretion of acid. The most commonly carried out surgical procedure is a Nissen fundoplication. This procedure in simple terms means wrapping the stomach around the oesophagus to change the anatomical angle and neurogenic reflex mechanisms. The aim is to prevent acid being refluxed from the stomach back into the oesophagus.

Dental Erosion

The role of GORD in dental erosion has been widely reported in the dental literature. Regurgitated acid entering the mouth causes dental erosion. The pattern of the erosion is similar to other conditions involving stomach juice such as eating disorders, rumination and chronic alcoholism. Since the acidity in the stomach may be below pH 1, frequent regurgitation or vomiting will erode teeth.

The evidence associating GORD and dental erosion comes from two main areas, patients presenting with symptoms of GORD who are then found to have dental erosion and patients presenting with dental erosion who are then found to have GORD.

Medical Evidence
The relationship between dental erosion and GORD has been investigated in children and adults. One of the first investigations of the association between

dental erosion and GORD was carried out by Jarvinen et al. [6]. They diagnosed GORD by using endoscopy to assess oesophagitis in 20 patients. Typically, in disease the appearance of the mucosa is reddened and inflamed and in chronic disease the lumen begins to close causing dysphagia. Dental erosion was assessed in the 20 oesophagitis patients by grading each tooth surface numerically using a tooth wear index. In the study group, 4 patients were found to have dental erosion. They concluded that patients diagnosed with GORD had a higher risk of developing dental erosion. Meurman et al. [7] carried out a similar study but included a larger group of 117 Finnish patients referred with symptoms of GORD. Dental erosion was reported to involve 24% of tooth surfaces. The authors concluded that severe reflux disease of long duration was more likely to cause dental erosion than milder forms. Aine et al. [48] reported the case results of 17 children with confirmed GORD and 2 children with dental erosion in whom this condition led to the diagnosis of GORD. They found that almost all children with pathological GOR had dental erosion of some type but the severity varied.

Moazzez et al. [9] in a study on patients referred to a gastroenterological clinic with symptoms of reflux assessed their tooth wear and compared the results to a control group. Tooth wear was assessed using the Smith and Knight Tooth Wear Index [49]. Tooth wear involving dentine was more prevalent in patients complaining of symptoms of GORD and those diagnosed as having GORD following 24-h pH monitoring than a control group. Patients with poorer salivary buffering capacity than controls and those complaining of hoarseness had lower salivary flow rate than controls. Therefore, the subjects were not only more likely to develop dental erosion they also had extra-oesophageal symptoms of reflux. This association is an interesting one and raises the possibility that once reflux passes through the UOS it can affect not only the teeth but also the surrounding structures including the larynx.

Another study by the same authors investigated with 24-h ambulatory pH monitoring at 4 sites along the oesophagus in patients complaining of extra-oesophageal reflux (including dental erosion, hoarseness, chronic coughs). The authors reported that the severity of reflux above the UOS was correlated to the severity of dental erosion, particularly on the palatal surfaces [50].

Dental Evidence

There is evidence from dental patients who are subsequently assessed for reflux disease. Gudmundsson et al. [13] measured oral pH and distal oesophageal pH in 14 patients with dental erosion. Dental erosion was graded as mild or severe. Oesophageal pH was measured at 5 cm above the LOS using an antimony pH electrode and 21% of patients were found to have pathological GORD and extended periods of lowered oral pH were recorded but the two did not coincide. The authors concluded that the erosion was a result of reduced salivary buffering capacity rather than GORD.

Schroeder et al. [10] in a small study of 12 patients with dental erosion investigated reflux using ambulatory 24-h oesophageal pH monitoring. Ten of the 12 dental patients were diagnosed with reflux disease but no relationship was reported between saliva and tooth wear. The authors also assessed the presence of dental erosion in a separate group of 30 patients with reflux disease as assessed by 24-h pH measurement. Twelve of 30 patients also had dental erosion. The authors separated the results into distal (near the stomach) and proximal reflux (near the UOS) and found that patients with proximal reflux had 7% of their teeth affected as opposed to those with distal reflux who had 3% of their teeth affected.

In a controlled study, Bartlett et al. [8] investigated 36 patients with palatal dental erosion. The results were compared to 10 subjects without tooth wear or symptoms of GORD. Oral pH was measured simultaneously. Twenty-three (64%) patients were found to have GORD and of these 16 were found to have GOR symptoms whilst the remaining 7 did not complain of any symptoms. The term 'silent refluxers' was used to describe these patients. The hypothesis in these patients suggested that patients with chronic reflux might have higher than normal pain thresholds or become unresponsive to pain. In addition, in this study a statistically significant relationship was observed between the low pH in the distal oesophagus and the pH in the mouth.

More recently, Gregory-Head et al. [51] reported a study comparing levels of tooth wear in 20 patients with symptoms of GORD compared to a group of controls. Ten of the patient group were diagnosed with GORD. Tooth wear was assessed using a tooth wear index and GORD was diagnosed using 24-h pH monitoring. GORD patients had significantly higher tooth wear scores compared with control subjects.

These tests assessed the presence of acid with the oesophagus. However, the efficiency of the oesophagus in moving fluids is important. Manometry measures the efficiency of the oesophagus in transporting fluids and is used indirectly to assess the capacity of the oesophagus to prevent reflux. One controlled study measured the motility of patients presenting with dental erosion. The authors reported that whilst the LOS sphincter pressure was normal, the motility of the oesophagus was abnormal compared to the controls. The assumption being that poor oesophageal motility led to the development of reflux and ultimately to dental erosion [52]. It is clear that dental erosion and GORD are related. However, the question still remains that why some people with GORD suffer from dental erosion and others not.

Table 3. Eating disorders

Anorexia	Bulimia
Mainly females	Mainly females
Low self-image	Low self-image
Western society	Western society
Compulsive	Compulsive
Intelligent	Intelligent
Early adolescence	Late adolescence
Dietary restriction	Binge/purging
Low body weight	Normal body weight
Low metabolic rate	Electrolyte imbalance
Minimal drug use	Drug and alcohol abuse

Eating Disorders

An eating disorder can be defined as a persistent avoidance of food or eating behaviour which impairs physical or psychosocial function and is not related to other medical conditions [53]. The two closely linked disorders are anorexia and bulimia nervosa (table 3). Eating disorders have been described by the Eating Disorders Association as the 'outward expression of deep psychological and emotional turmoil, with sufferers turning to food and eating as a means of expressing their difficulties'. Anorexia nervosa is the refusal to maintain normal body weight. Bulimia is derived from the Greek, meaning ox hunger and characterised by binge eating followed by behavioural responses aimed at avoiding body weight gain.

Anorexia Nervosa

The literal meaning is 'a nervous loss of appetite' and is derived from the Greek word orexis or appetite [53]. There are four basic features common to most anorexics: severe weight loss (less than 85% of normal body weight), amenorrhoea, psychological disturbances and increased activity. But the most important feature is a relentless pursuit of thinness [53]. This pursuit continues despite being thin. Suffers continue to avoid food because of an altered body image driving them to further food restriction. There is an understanding that anorexia has two clinical subtypes: restrictive and binge/purge. The former pursue their goals through dietary restriction whilst the latter aid this through purging and laxatives. The distinction between the subtypes can be blurred as sufferers pass from one form to another.

The annual incidence of anorexia in Britain has been estimated at between 0.6 and 1.6 per 100,000 of the whole population [54]. This is a socio-cultural disease affecting white, upper and middle class women between the ages of 12 and 30 years [55, 56]. It is an overwhelming disease of Westernised Industrial societies and is ten times more common in females than males [57].

This disease may begin abruptly as a single circumscribed episode or develop gradually over many months or even over a number of years [58]. A person with a low self-esteem and compulsive behaviour who strives for perfection is more likely to develop the disease. Anorexia is found in intelligent, highly motivated individuals often with over-protective parents [59]. They are often isolated and restrictive in their behaviour with an underlying fear of adult responsibilities and use self-denial as an escape from growing up [60].

The aetiology of anorexia nervosa is known to have a number of influencing factors including genetic, temperament/personality, developmental and sociocultural influences [53, 59, 61]. Family and twin studies suggest that a strong genetic component is important in anorexia [62] but the origin of the heritable feature is unknown. Personality traits include perfectionism and obsessional behaviour which can occur alongside the fear of weight gain. Developmental factors occur during early adolescence and may be related to onset of puberty [53]. Psychological stress may play a role in precipitating the condition. Finally, the impact of modern society and its reliance on body image may also have an important role in the development of the condition. It is a secretive disease which may pass through periods of exacerbation and quiescence. In some patients, it is difficult to distinguish between anorexia and bulimia nervosa. Almost all anorexics deny the illness and refuse therapy and around 25% of the serious cases die of medical complications [56].

Clinically, the condition can be diagnosed by someone with less than 85% of their ideal or normal body weight. Initially, anorexics may start a gradual transition with limitations to high-calorie foods, later meat avoidance and finally reliance on 'safe foods' without any calorific gain. The continual weight loss has medical implications with poor concentration, decline of interest, and social avoidance. With increasing severity, symptoms recorded are bradycardia, hair loss, low body temperature, dry skin, and carotenodermia (yellow–orange skin) on the palms and soles of the feet. Other medical problems such as gastrointestinal- (decreased gastric emptying and constipation) and kidney-related disorders (increased blood urea concentrations, renal calculi) as well as osteoporosis have also been described.

Overactivity is a common feature of anorexia and considered by some to be an essential component [53]. It may take on various forms and exercise combined with dietary restriction has a very profound impact on weight loss. This occurs with an altered drive to eat with avoidance and control of hunger. The altered body image distorts their awareness of self despite obvious changes to those around them. These changes in body image occur with depressive symptoms in the acutely underweight individuals [63]. Treatment of anorexia is multi-level and multi-disciplinary. Hospital-based treatment includes in-patient and out-patient care.

Bulimia

The term was derived from the Greek word bous and limos literally meaning 'ox hunger'. The condition was first noted in the late 1970s by Russell [64]. The identifying feature is binge eating with an excessive amount of food with a subjective loss of control [53]. Binge eating is associated with behaviour aimed to avoid weight gain most often through self-induced vomiting. The diagnosis is made when binge eating and vomiting occurs more than twice a week for at least 3 months. Body weight for bulimic is normal and if it drops then anorexia becomes part of the condition. Some characteristics involve subtyping into purging and non-purging variants. Among the purging types metabolic disturbances are more common with electrolyte imbalance and lower body weight.

It is difficult to find reliable data for the prevalence of bulimia in the UK. Patients with bulimia are normally slightly older than anorexics, typically in their early 20s, while late-onset anorexia nervosa affects adolescents. Some estimates are about 1–3% of females [65]. The male to female ratio is 1:10 [53]. Dieting usually precedes disease onset although some report binge eating prior to the onset [53].

Many of the risk factors identified in anorexia are common to bulimia and some merging of the conditions is known to occur. Early critical comments about weight can be identified as precursors of the condition. Unlike anorexia there is more of a tendency for self-abuse such as alcohol, drugs and self-mutilation [66]. The clinical features of the condition involve use of vomiting, laxatives and diuretics to control body weight. As the condition evolves, the appeal of food reduces and binge eating and purging increases. This may be associated with low feeling or self and depression. Some bulimics identify 'forbidden foods' which provoke them to lose control and are contrasted to 'safe foods' which allow them to maintain control [53].

Treatment for the condition is generally unsatisfactory. Efforts are directed at regaining physical health, reducing the symptoms and improving self-esteem [58]. Medication can be used together with psychological counselling. Some larger hospitals have joint clinics with psychologists, therapists, gastroenterologists and other specialists present to co-ordinate and supervise the patient's management and occasionally dentists are also present.

A relatively new condition has been described called Binge-Eating Disorder. It is characterised by recurrent binge-eating episodes of more than

2 days a week for 6 months. Eating is quicker than normal and continues until the person is uncomfortably full and occurs in the absence of hunger and often when alone [57]. Unlike bulimia, it does not involve purging or vomiting. It might also be classified as bulimia non-purging type.

Dental Implications

The oral status of patients with eating disorders has been assessed in several studies [67]. It is evident that a common presenting feature is erosion of the palatal (lingual) surfaces of the upper anterior teeth but also the posterior teeth as well. The appearance of palatal erosion was first described as periomylolysis [68]. The main differences between eating disorders appears to be that severe palatal and moderate buccal erosion is apparent in virtually all those who vomit, but rare in non-vomiting patients. Those suffers using purging to rid themselves of food have an increased risk of developing erosion. The main support from this observation comes from two early papers from Scandinavia [67, 69]. However, both studies recognised that a contribution from the subject's diet, which included acidic foods and drinks, was possible. Although, it might be expected that vomiting and erosion are directly related, one study observed the contrary. The authors reported that the frequency, duration and total number of vomiting episodes was not directly related to erosion [55]. The same authors did not find a relationship between level of erosion and frequency of vomiting. Both that and another study reported relationships between erosion and those reporting self-induced vomiting [41]. This apparent dilemma suggests that other factors are involved with the development of erosion. For those with non-vomiting and restrictive diets, particularly those with anorexia, are less likely to develop erosion but the risk still exists later in life. In addition, because of the complex nature of the condition those who have controlled their eating disorder may still retain a higher risk of continuing dental erosion because of the link between it and GOR.

The distribution of erosion is on the palatal surfaces of the upper anterior teeth [41]. This study also reported more erosion on the occlusal and buccal surfaces of the lower posterior teeth and this difference was independent of whether vomiting occurred or not. This might be explained with the increased consumption of acidic drinks but it is not clear [70]. But chronic suffers, for 5 years or more, are more likely to develop more widespread erosion [70]. Milosevic and Slade [55] also recognised that prolonged vomiting over extensive periods of time increased the risk of developing erosion. Rytömaa et al. [71] compared the incidence of dental erosion in a group of 35 bulimics and compared the results to 105 controls and also reported severe erosion in patients compared with a similar group of controls. A recent study from Australia investigating 30 patients with an eating disorder and compared their tooth wear to a matched control group [72]. After examining their study casts, the authors reported that those with the eating disorders had more erosion than the controls. Overall, palatal dental erosion is commonly found in vomiting eating disorders.

An increased risk of caries has also been reported but the association is unclear [73]. In Hellstrom's [67] paper there were no differences between vomiting and non-vomiting subjects whilst another reported less caries in anorexics [69] but neither study compared their results to a control group. Other workers have not found any association [41, 55, 70]. Overall, there seems to be little agreement on whether caries is increased or decreased in eating disorders and may reflect the changing and merging of signs and symptoms in these subjects.

Saliva might be expected to be important particularly with self-induced vomiting because of the autonomic nervous system control of the process. Also changes to electrolyte balance seen in vomiting might be expected to have an impact on saliva. Rytömaa et al. [71] reported decreased salivary flow rate in their study of bulimics. Another study of 35 subjects with eating disorders also reported decreased unstimulated salivary flow rate and suggested that tests of salivary flow may serve as an indicator of the risk of progression of erosion [74]. Normal salivary flow has been reported in non-vomiting anorexics and bulimics [75]. Other workers have reported significantly lower rates of salivary flow in their study of vomiting bulimics with and without dental erosion [76]. These workers also measured bicarbonate ion levels and observed reduced levels irrespective of vomiting but increased viscosity in the subjects with erosion. This may reflect the changes in electrolyte balance found in the vomiting groups. There are difficulties in measuring saliva as the testing methods are not universally accepted nor are they particularly accurate. Finally, an observation that parotid enlargement occurs in bulimia has been reported by a number of authors [77, 78].

Chronic Alcoholism

Chronic alcoholism is a serious condition with potentially life-threatening complications. Some alcoholics present with dental erosion. The pattern of wear suggests that the source of the acid is regurgitated stomach juice. Attrition due to bruxism has also been reported in alcoholics [79]. Chronic alcoholism is thought to affect 10% of the population although this figure overestimates the probable prevalence [80]. Alcohol can result in gastritis and provoke GOR [81]. Alcoholics also have poor diet control and tend to eat more acidic foods and drinks. Tooth wear has been found to be more prevalent in studies comparing alcoholics to controls [40, 82]. In this study of 31 patients with chronic alcoholism, tooth wear was frequently observed on the palatal surfaces of the upper anterior teeth.

Rumination

Rumination is a rare but interesting condition that can cause severe dental erosion. The pattern of erosion in these patients is similar to other conditions where the acid is regurgitated from the stomach, such as eating disorders. Subjects regurgitate their food which can be solid or liquid, sometimes re-chew the food and then swallow again. They repeatedly raise their intra-abdominal pressure after meals and regurgitation occurs when one of these compressions coincides with swallowing and the associated relaxation of the lower oesophageal sphincter [83]. Rumination occurs commonly in people with learning difficulties but it can affect other members of the population.

It has been reported that rumination may be more common than was previously thought. It has also been suggested that it affects highly intelligent, professional people [84]. The pathophysiology of rumination is poorly understood and has been incompletely studied. It is generally considered to be a psychological disorder although it has also been suggested that patients might suffer from GORD. Patients often find it embarrassing to admit to the condition and the prevalence might be higher than was first thought.

The pattern of dental erosion is similar to other intrinsic causes with the first signs developing on the palatal surfaces of the upper incisors and if the condition continues to involve other tooth surfaces. Because the gastric juice is forced into the mouth just after feeding it is generally quite acidic and the resulting erosion is normally severe.

Pregnancy and Other Causes

Pregnancy is not strictly recognised as an eating disorder, but the hormonal changes are well known to affect eating habits during the term. Unusual eating habits can develop during pregnancy [39] but these tend to be temporary and return to normal after the birth. Unexpectedly, anorexics or bulimics may actually improve whilst being pregnant [85]. Vomiting during pregnancy can occur especially during the first trimester and may cause further erosion. There is also increased reflux in pregnancy.

Conclusion

Intrinsic causes of dental erosion involve stomach acids entering the mouth. These strong acids erode the enamel and dentine normally starting on the palatal surfaces of the upper anterior teeth. The strength of the acid often results in severe erosion resulting in significant loss of enamel and dentine. As the condition progresses the damage to teeth becomes more widespread.

The conditions associated with the movement of the acid from the stomach to the mouth are generally related to reflux disease. The relationship between GOR and dental erosion has been well documented. The association has been investigated in patients presenting with GOR and in those presenting with dental erosion. An association between GOR and dental erosion has been found in both groups.

The association of eating disorders and dental erosion has also been well reported. Persistent vomiting has been observed to cause dental erosion and is commonly found in patients with eating disorders.

Gastric causes of dental erosion are probably relatively uncommon but when they do occur, the damage to teeth is often severe and time consuming to treat.

References

1   Bartlett DW, Coward PY: Comparison of erosive potential of gastric juice and a carbonated drink in vitro. J Oral Rehabil 2001;28:1045–1047.
2   Kidd EAM, Smith BGN: Toothwear histories: a sensitive issue. Dent Update 1993;20:174–178.
3   Smith BGN, Knight JK: A comparison of patterns of tooth wear with aetiological factors. Br Dent J 1984;157:16–19.
4   Lussi A, Schaffner M, Holtz P, Suter P: Dental erosion in a population of Swiss adults. Community Dent Oral Epidemiol 1991;19:286–290.
5   Jarvinen V, Rytomaa II, Heinonen OP: Risk factors in dental erosion. J Dent Res 1991;70:942–947.
6   Jarvinen V, Meurman JH, Hyvarinen H, Rytomaa I, Murtomaa H: Dental erosion and upper gastrointestinal disorders. Oral Surg Oral Med Oral Pathol 1988;65:298–303.
7   Meurman JH, Toskala J, Nuutinen P, Klemetti E: Oral and dental manifestations in gastroesophageal reflux disease. Oral Surg Oral Med Oral Pathol 1994;78:583–589.
8   Bartlett DW, Evans DF, Anggiansah A, Smith BGN: A study of the association between gastro-oesophageal reflux and palatal dental erosion. Br Dent J 1996;181:125–131.
9   Moazzez R, Anggiansah A, Bartlett DW: Dental erosion, gastro-oesophageal reflux disease and saliva: how are they related? J Dent 2004;32:489–494.
10 Schroeder PL, Filler SJ, Ramirez B, Lazarchik DA, Vaezi MF, Richter JE: Dental erosion and acid reflux disease. Ann Intern Med 1995;122:809–815.
11 O'Sullivan EA, Curzon ME, Roberts GJ, Milla PJ, Stringer MD: Gastroesophageal reflux in children and its relationship to erosion of primary and permanent teeth. Eur J Oral Sci 1998;106:765–769.
12 Gregory-Head BL, Curtis DA: Erosion caused by gastroesophageal reflux: diagnostic considerations. J Prosthodont 1997;6:278–285.
13 Gudmundsson K, Kristleifsson G, Theodors A, Holbrook WP: Tooth erosion, gastroesophageal reflux, and salivary buffer capacity. Oral Surg Oral Med Oral Pathol 1995;79:185–189.
14 Bartlett DW, Ricketts DNJ, Fisher NL: Management of the short clinical crown by indirect restorations. Dent Update 1997;24:431–436.
15 Bartlett DW: Adapting crown preparations to adhesive materials. Dent Update 2000;27:460–463.
16 Meyer GW, Austin RM, Brady CE III, Castell DO: Muscle anatomy of the human esophagus. J Clin Gastroenterol 1986;8:131–134.
17 Peters FT, Kleibeuker JH: Barrett's oesophagus and carcinoma: recent insights into its development and possible prevention. Scand J Gastroenterol Suppl 1993;200:59–64.
18 Buthpitiya AG, Stroud D, Russell CO: Pharyngeal pump and esophageal transit. Dig Dis Sci 1987;32:1244–1248.

19 Richter JE, Wu WC, Johns DN, Blackwell JN, Nelson JL, Castell JA, et al: Esophageal manometry in 95 healthy adult volunteers: variability of pressures with age and frequency of 'abnormal' contractions. Dig Dis Sci 1987;32:583–592.

20 Johnson LF, DeMeester TR: Twenty four hour pH monitoring of the distal esophagus. Am J Gastroenterol 1974;62:325–332.

21 Benjamin SB, Richter JE, Cordova CM, Knuff TE, Castell DO: Prospective manometric evaluation with pharmacologic provocation of patients with suspected esophageal motility dysfunction. Gastroenterol Int 1983;84:893–901.

22 Janssens J, Vantrappen G, Ghillebert G: 24-hour recording of esophageal pressure and pH in patients with noncardiac chest pain. Gastroenterology 1986;90:1978–1984.

23 Vantrappen G, Janssens J: Pathophysiology and treatment of gastro-oesophageal reflux disease. Scand J Gastroenterol 1989;24(suppl):7–12.

24 Wilson JA, Heading RC: The proximal sphincters; in Kumar D, Wingate D (eds): An Illustrated Guide to Gastrointestinal Motility, ed 2. London, Churchill-Livingstone, 1993, pp 357–372.

25 Chandra A, Moazzez R, Bartlett DW, Anggiansah A, Owen WJ: A review of the atypical manifestations of gastroesophageal reflux disease. Int J Clin Pract 2004;58:41–48.

26 Hennesey TPJ, Cuschieri A, Bennett JR: Reflux Oesophagitis, ed 1. London, Butterworth, 1989.

27 Castell DO, Holtz A: Gastroesophageal reflux. Postgrad Med 1989;86:141–148.

28 Nebel OT, Fornes MF, Castell DO: Symptomatic gastroesophageal reflux: incidence and precipitating factors. Dig Dis 1976;21:953–956.

29 Bennett JR: Heartburn and gastro-oesophageal reflux. Br J Clin Pract 1991;45:273–277.

30 Bartlett DW, Evans DF, Smith BGN: The relationship between gastro-oesophageal reflux disease and dental erosion (review). J Oral Rehabil 1996;23:289–297.

31 Kitchen LI, Castell DO: Rationale and efficacy of conservative therapy for gastroesophageal reflux disease. Arch Intern Med 1991;151:448–454.

32 Irwin RS, French CL, Curley FJ, Zawacki JK, Bennett FM: Chronic cough due to gastroesophageal reflux. Chest 1993;104:1511–1517.

33 Chernow B, Johnson LF, Janowitz WR, Castell DO: Pulmonary aspiration as a consequence of gastroesophageal reflux: a diagnostic approach. Dig Dis Sci 1979;24:839–844.

34 Irwin RS, Madison JM: Anatomical diagnostic protocol in evaluating chronic cough with specific reference to gastroesophageal reflux disease. Am J Med 2000;108(suppl 4a):126S–130S.

35 Irwin RS, Richter JE: Gastroesophageal reflux and chronic cough. Am J Gastroenterol 2000;95(suppl):S9–S14.

36 Field SK: Gastroesophageal reflux and respiratory symptoms. Chest 1999;116:843.

37 Field SK, Underwood M, Brant R, Cowie RL: Prevalence of gastroesophageal reflux symptoms in asthma. Chest 1996;109:316–322.

38 Field SK: Underlying mechanisms of respiratory symptoms with esophageal acid when there is no evidence of airway response. Am J Med 2001;111(suppl 8A):37S–40S.

39 McLoughlin IJ, Hassanyeh F: Pica in a patient with anorexia nervosa. Br J Psychiatry 1990;156: 568–570.

40 Robb ND: Dental erosion in patients with chronic alcoholism. J Dent 1989;17:219–221.

41 Robb ND, Smith BG, Geidrys-Leeper E: The distribution of erosion in the dentitions of patients with eating disorders. Br Dent J 1995;178:171–175.

42 Smit CF, van Leeuwen JA, Mathus-Vliegen LM, Devriese PP, Semin A, Tan J, et al: Gastropharyngeal and gastroesophageal reflux in globus and hoarseness. Arch Otolaryngol Head Neck Surg 2000;126:827–830.

43 Koufman JA: Laryngopharyngeal reflux is different from classic gastroesophageal reflux disease. Ear Nose Throat J 2002;81(suppl 2):7–9.

44 Vitale GC, Cheadle WG, Patel B, Sadek SA: The effect of alcohol on nocturnal gastroesophageal reflux. JAMA 1987;258:2077–2079.

45 Kraus BB, Jane W, Sinclair PA, Castell DO: Gastroesophageal reflux in runners. Ann Intern Med 1990;112:429–433.

46 Hirsch DP, Mathus-Vliegen EM, Dagli U, Tytgat GN, Boeckxstaens GE: Effect of prolonged gastric distention on lower esophageal sphincter function and gastroesophageal reflux. Am J Gastroenterol 2003;98:1696–1704.

Intrinsic Causes of Erosion

47 Klauser AG, Heinrich C, Schindlbeck NE, Muller-Lissner SA: Is long-term esophageal monitoring of clinical value? Am J Gastroenterol 1989;84:362–366.

48 Aine L, Baer M, Maki M: Dental erosions caused by gastroesophageal reflux disease in children. J Dent Child 1993;60:210–214.

49 Smith BGN, Knight JK: An index for measuring the wear of teeth. Br Dent J 1984;156:435–438.

50 Moazzez R, Anggiansah A, Bartlett DW: The association of high reflux and tooth wear. Caries Res 2005; in press.

51 Gregory-Head BL, Curtis DA, Kim L, Cello J: Evaluation of dental erosion in patients with gastroesophageal reflux disease. J Prosthet Dent 2000;83:675–680.

52 Bartlett DW, Evans DF, Anggiansah A, Smith BGN: The role of the esophagus in dental erosion. Oral Surg Oral Med Oral Pathol Oral Radiol Endod 1999;89:312–315.

53 Klein DA, Walsh BT: Eating disorders: clinical features and pathophysiology. Physiol Behav 2004;81:359–374.

54 Kendal RE, Hall DJ, Babigan HM: The epidemiology of anorexia nervosa. Psychol Med 1973;3: 200–203.

55 Milosevic A, Slade PD: The orodental status of anorexics and bulimics. Br Dent J 1989;167:66–70.

56 Jensen OE, Featherstone JDB, Stege P: Chemical and physical oral findings in a case of anorexia nervosa and bulimia. J Oral Pathol Med 1987;16:399–402.

57 Williamson DA, Martin CK, Stewart T: Psychological aspects of eating disorders. Best Pract Res Clin Gastroenterol 2004;18:1073–1088.

58 Herzog DB, Copeland PM: Eating disorders. N Engl J Med 1985;313:295–303.

59 Knewitz JL, Drisko CL: Anorexia nervosa and bulimia: a review. Compendium 1988;9:244–247.

60 Andrews FFH: Dental erosion due to anorexia nervosa and bulimia. Br Dent J 1982;152:89–90.

61 Knewitz JL, Drisko CL: Anorexia nervosa and bulimia: a review. Compendium 1992;11:244–247.

62 Klump KL, Kaye WH, Strober M: The evolving genetic foundations of eating disorders. Child Adolesc Psychiatr Clin N Am 2001;24:215–225.

63 Kaye WH: Anorexia nervosa, obsessional behavior, and serotonin. Psychopharmacol Bull 1997;33:335–344.

64 Russell G: Bulimia nervosa: an ominous variant of anorexia nervosa. Psychol Med 1979;9:429–448.

65 Kendler KS, MacLean C, Neale M, Kessler R, Heath A, Eaves L: The genetic epidemiology of bulimia nervosa. Am J Psychiatry 1991;148:1627–1637.

66 Lilenfeld LR, Stein D, Bulik CM, Strober M, Plotnicov K, Pollice C, et al: Personality traits among currently eating disordered, recovered and never ill first-degree female relatives of bulimic and control women. Psychol Med 2000;30:1399–1410.

67 Hellstrom I: Oral complications in anorexia nervosa. Scand J Dent Res 1977;85:71–86.

68 Holst JJ, Lange F: A contribution towards the genesis of tooth wasting from non-mechanical causes. Acta Odontol Scand 1939;26:396.

69 Hurst PS, Lacey LH, Crisp AH: Teeth, vomiting and diet: a study of the dental characteristics of seventeen anorexia nervosa patients. Postgrad Med J 1977;53:298–305.

70 Scheutzel P: Etiology of dental erosion – intrinsic factors. Eur J Oral Sci 1996;104:178–190.

71 Rytömaa I, Järvinen V, Kanerva R, Heinonen OP: Bulimia and tooth erosion. Acta Odontol Scand 1998;56:36–40.

72 Valena V, Young WG: Dental erosion patterns from intrinsic acid regurgitation and vomiting. Aust Dent J 2002;47:106–115.

73 Milosevic A: Eating disorders and the dentist. Br Dent J 1999;186:109–113.

74 Ohrn R, Angmar-Mansson B: Oral status of 35 subjects with eating disorders: a 1-year study. Eur J Oral Sci 2000;108:275–280.

75 Touyz SW, Liew VP, Tseng P, Frisken K, Williams H, Beumont PJ: Oral and dental complications in dieting disorders. Int J Eat Disord 1993;14:341–347.

76 Milosevic A, Dawson LJ: Salivary factors in vomiting bulimics with and without pathological tooth wear. Caries Res 1996;30:361–366.

77 Levin PA, Falko JM, Dixon K: Benign parotid enlargement in bulimia. Ann Intern Med 1980;93:827–829.

78 Hasler JF: Parotid enlargement: a presenting sign in anorexia nervosa. Oral Surg Oral Med Oral Pathol 1982;53:567–573.

79   King WH, Tucker KM: Dental problems of alcoholic and nonalcoholic psychiatric patients. Q J Stud Alcohol 1973;34:1208–1211.
80   Christen AG: Dentistry and the alcoholic patient. Dent Clin N Am 1983;27:341–361.
81   Gottfried EB, Korsten MA, Lieber CS: Alcohol-induced gastric and duodenol lesions in man. Am J Gastroenterol 1978;70:587–592.
82   Robb ND, Smith BGN: Prevalence of pathological tooth wear in patients with chronic alcoholism. Br Dent J 1990;169:367–369.
83   Levine DF, Wingate DL, Pfeffer JM, Butcher P: Habitual rumination: a benign disorder. Br Med J 1983;287:255–256.
84   Gilmour AG, Beckett HA: The voluntary reflux phenomenon. Br Dent J 1994;175:368–372.
85   Fairburn CG, Stein A, Jones R: Eating habits and eating disorders during pregnancy. Psychosom Med 1992;54:665–672.
86   DeMeester TR, Johnson LF, Joseph GJ, Toscano MS, Hall AW, Skinner DB: Patterns of gastroesophageal reflux in health and disease. Ann Surg 1976;184:459–469.

David Bartlett
Department of Prosthodontics, GKT Dental Institute
Floor 25, Guy's Tower, St. Thomas' Street
London Bridge, London SE1 9RT (UK)

Lussi A (ed): Dental Erosion.
Monogr Oral Sci. Basel, Karger, 2006, vol 20, pp 140–151

....

Dental Erosion in Children

A. Lussi, T. Jaeggi

Department of Preventive, Restorative and Pediatric Dentistry,
School of Dental Medicine, University of Bern, Bern, Switzerland

Abstract

Erosive tooth wear in children is a common condition. The overlapping of erosion with mechanical forces like attrition or abrasion is probably in deciduous teeth more pronounced than in permanent teeth. Early erosive damage to the permanent teeth may compromise the dentition for the entire lifetime and require extensive restorative procedures. Therefore, early diagnosis of the condition and adequate preventive measures are of importance. Knowledge of the etiological factors for erosive tooth wear is a prerequisite for such measures. In children and adolescents (like in adults) extrinsic and intrinsic factors or a combination of them are possible reasons for the condition. Such factors are frequent and extensive consumption of erosive foodstuffs and drinks, the intake of medicaments (asthma), gastro-esophageal reflux (a case history is discussed) or vomiting. But also behavioral factors like unusual eating and drinking habits, the consumption of designer drugs and socio-economic aspects are of importance.

We here present an overview of dental erosion with an emphasis on aspects of topics not covered in other chapters.

Tooth wear is a cumulative multifactorial process, which begins following eruption of the teeth and is to a certain degree considered a physiologic condition. What we consider an acceptable amount of wear is dependent on the lifespan of the teeth and, therefore, is much shorter for deciduous compared to permanent teeth. However, erosive damage to the permanent teeth occurring in early childhood (fig. 1) may compromise the dentition for the child's entire lifetime and may require repeated expensive restoration. Therefore, it is important that early diagnosis of the tooth wear process is achieved and adequate preventive measures are undertaken.

For a dentist, it is important to detect the main etiological factor of tooth wear in order to implement the required preventive measures. A very early sign

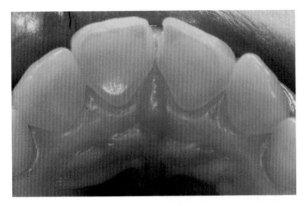

Fig. 1. Erosive tooth wear of an 8-year-old boy on the palatal surfaces of the upper permanent incisors.

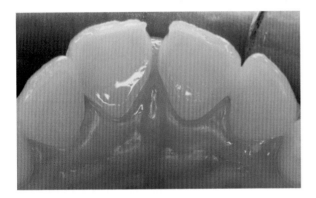

Fig. 2. Same case as figure 1 after treatment of the hypersensitive palatal surfaces with a sealant.

of dental erosion is the silky glazed appearance of the enamel. Common sites for dental erosion in primary teeth are the occlusal aspects of the molars and the palatal surfaces of the upper incisors (figs. 1, 3, 4) [1, 2].

Deciduous teeth are smaller than permanent teeth, the enamel is thinner, and there are morphological differences compared to permanent teeth. Therefore, the erosive process reaches the dentine earlier and leads to an advanced lesion after a shorter exposure to acids, compared with permanent teeth [3].

While in vitro studies investigating erosion in deciduous teeth found the enamel of primary teeth to be softer than that of permanent teeth, the in vitro susceptibility of these teeth to softening revealed conflicting results, and

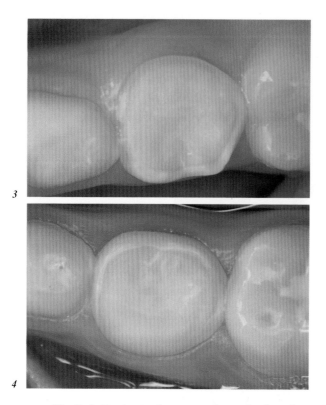

Fig. 3, 4. Erosive tooth wear on the occlusal surfaces of the lower primary molars. Advanced erosions with involvement of dentine are visible. The condition is distinct and reaches both the buccal and oral aspects.

demonstrated either a higher susceptibility of deciduous or permanent enamel to erosion. Amaechi et al. [4] examined the substance loss of deciduous and permanent teeth after immersion in orange juice. They found a 1.5 times greater progression of erosive lesions into the enamel of the primary dentition compared to that of the permanent dentition [4]. In contrast to these findings, Hunter et al. [5] measured only small differences in the susceptibility to erosion of deciduous and permanent teeth. Maupomé et al. [6] investigated the effect of a cola drink on deciduous and permanent enamel incorporating an early salivary pellicle. When primary and permanent teeth were exposed to acidic beverages, no statistically significant differences were found in the rate of surface softening for both tooth types. In another study, 60 primary and 60 permanent human teeth were immersed for 3 min in 12 different beverages and foodstuffs. Surface microhardness was measured before and after exposure.

Initial (baseline) surface microhardness was lower for primary teeth than for permanent teeth. In both primary and permanent teeth, no statistically significant differences in the decrease of microhardness were found for the two enamel types. Overall decrease was 27 ± 17 KHN (mean $\pm$ SD) for primary and 26 ± 16 KHN for permanent teeth. The same pattern was found when enamel was immersed for 6 min in different beverages and foodstuffs [7, 8]. Lippert et al. [9] used nanoindentation combined with atomic force microscopy to investigate the erosive effect of four different drinks on enamel at early stages in vitro. In this short-term experiment, deciduous enamel was not found to be more susceptible to erosion than permanent enamel. In another study, a longer immersion time of up to 30 min and a more aggressive softening solution (2% citric acid, pH 2.1, 37°C) was tested. Here, the microhardness measurements showed that enamel surface hardness decreased proportionately with increased time of immersion, in all tooth specimen groups. When permanent teeth were compared to deciduous teeth, the differences in microhardness were found to be statistically significant, with deciduous teeth being softer than the permanent teeth, both at baseline and after immersion in acid [10].

From the above studies, it seems that the increased susceptibility of deciduous enamel to erosion does not appear to occur in the initial phase, but rather over time and/or with increasing softening power of the acid. This is of importance to the clinician given the reduced dimension of the deciduous dentition and the continuously increasing intake of soft drinks by children. In addition, softer enamel such as the enamel of deciduous teeth is more prone to abrasion [11], which may explain the clinical picture often seen in children with significant tooth surface loss. The overlapping of erosion with attrition and/or abrasion is probably more pronounced in deciduous than in permanent teeth.

Extrinsic Factors

Diet

Diet has been the most extensively studied etiological factor in dental erosion, although systematic studies examining deciduous teeth are rare [12]. Excessive consumption of acidic (soft) drinks and foodstuffs is the most important extrinsic factor for dental erosion [13–15].

Data of the European and international trade associations representing the nonalcoholic beverages industry show a continuous increase of the consumption of nonalcoholic beverages in Europe in the last years [16]. Children and adolescents consume significant amounts of these mostly erosive beverages and therefore their risk of developing dental erosion is high. Soft drink intake in children is generally greater than in adults, but has a huge individual variation.

Forty-two percent of fruit drinks of the total consumption in Great Britain are consumed by children aged between 2 and 9 years [17]. In 1995, between 56 and 85% of schoolchildren in the USA consumed at least 1 soft drink daily, with the greatest amounts being ingested by adolescent males. Of this group, 20% consumed 4 or more servings daily [18, 19]. Assessment of erosive tooth wear in 14-year-old children (209 male, 209 female) in England revealed that over 80% regularly consumed soft drinks [20]. More than 10% had more than 3 intakes per day. There were statistically significant correlations between the prevalence of erosion and the consumption of soft drinks, carbonated beverages, alcoholic drinks, fresh fruits and others. The questionnaire data analysis also gave significant correlation between the consumption and frequency of milk, tea and yoghurt with erosion. These findings could be the expression of life-style rather than of a direct detrimental effect because milk, yoghurt and (black) tea do not produce erosion (see chapter 7.1.1 by Lussi, this vol, pp 77–99).

In a case-control study, standard salivary parameters were measured before and after soft drink intake in 30 children with erosive lesions and compared to those of 30 healthy children matched for sex. The results showed significant differences between the case and control children for salivary pH, flow rate, buffering capacity, maximum pH drop and minimum pH reached after soft drink intake. It was concluded that these factors are involved in dental erosion and that preventive care is mandatory for children who frequently drink these types of beverages [21]. It was also highlighted that administration of fruit juice in a feeding bottle leads to prolonged exposure to acidic pHs, especially if the feeding bottle is used as a comforter, e.g. at night [22]. In China, dental examinations carried out on 1,949 children aged 3–5 years revealed a statistically significant correlation between the presence of dental erosion and intake of fruit drink from a bottle or consumption of fruit drinks at bedtime. Furthermore, a significantly higher prevalence of erosion was found in children of a higher social class [23]. Prevalence data from a cross-sectional national study in the UK indicated that dietary associations with erosion are present, but weak [24]. In addition, in a sample of 418 14-year-olds, no statistically significant differences were found in the incidence of dental erosion between vegetarian and nonvegetarian children [25].

As is true for permanent teeth, frequent exposure to acidic juices and beverages can result in dental erosion in deciduous teeth. Based on the epidemiological studies in children and adults, and on case reports of children, acidic fruits and juices and acid beverages are most probably the principal cause of dental erosion in childhood. When this substance loss begins at a young age, there is a greater chance of losing tooth substance continuously over a lifetime, if no adequate preventive measures are performed. It can be stated that dietary factors represent the most important external risk factor for children to develop dental erosion.

Medicaments

The frequent use of acidic medications that come in direct contact with teeth has been identified as an etiological factor in dental erosion not only for adults but also for children and adolescents. Acetylsalicylic acid (aspirin) indicated for use by active juvenile rheumatoid arthritis sufferers is given at a dose of 90–130 mg/kg body weight [26]. Ascorbic acid (vitamin C) has been implicated in childhood dental erosion based on case reports [27]. Reports concerning the influence of asthma medication on dental erosion are controversial. In a case-control study, Al-Dlaigan et al. [28] compared three groups of children aged 11–18 years: 20 children with asthma requiring long-term medication, 20 children referred with dental erosion, and 20 children who were age- and sex-matched in the control group. There were significant differences in the prevalence of erosion between the three groups, with children with asthma requiring long-term medication having a higher prevalence than those of the control group [28]. Shaw et al. [29] examined and recorded the level of tooth wear in a random sample of 418 children from 12 secondary schools, the prevalence of asthma in this group was 16%. The amount of dental erosion in children with asthma was higher. In another survey, over 1,300 12-year-old children were examined for evidence of erosion then re-examined 2 years later. The presence of asthma was recorded on a self-completed questionnaire at the initial examination. It was found that tooth erosion was present in 59% of children with asthma and in 60% who were asthma free with no change over time. Eighty-eight percent of the drugs prescribed for treatment of asthma in this study had a pH which does not harm the teeth [30].

Behavioral, Biological and Socioeconomic Factors

The clinical expression of dental erosion is highly variable with some individuals experiencing total destruction of their teeth and others maintaining most of their tooth structure through a lifetime. Behavioral and biological factors are likely to account for some of the variability (see chapter 1 by Lussi, this vol, pp 1–8).

Case reports have linked erosion with abusive or unusual behaviors. Frequent and excessive consumption of specific dietary substances such as citrus fruits, lemon juice, orange juice, fruit squashes, cola-flavored soft drinks and citrus flavored drinks have all been implicated. Unusual eating, drinking and swallowing habits, e.g. holding an acid beverage in the mouth before swallowing, increase the contact time of an acidic substance with the teeth and thus the risk of erosion. The aim of a case-control study was to compare the diets of children with dental erosion with those who were caries-active or caries-free.

It showed that children with erosion drank acidic beverages significantly more frequently than children who either had caries or were caries-free [31]. Children with tooth erosion also drank milk or water significantly less often than the control groups and were more likely to have a swishing or holding habit associated with drinking. Fruit and vinegar consumption was higher in the erosion group, as was the intake of vitamin C supplements [31].

Bedtime consumption of acid beverages is also considered as a risk factor, especially for children. Several reports have suggested that the recent dramatic increase in consumption of acidic fruit juices, fruit drinks and carbonated beverages may be leading to a higher prevalence of erosion especially in young children and adolescents. The use of illegal designer drugs by teenagers at 'raves' has been associated with increased risk of erosion due to excessive consumption of acidic beverages [32].

The socioeconomic status of a population can also influence the occurrence for erosive tooth wear because of different eating and drinking and (perhaps) hygiene habits of these groups. Millward et al. [1] examined the prevalence of erosion of 178 4-year-old children and found more erosion in the higher socioeconomic groups. A significantly higher prevalence of erosion was found in children in China who had frequently consumed fruit drinks as a baby, and whose parents had a higher education level [23]. The reasons suggested for the increased erosion in the higher social class was a more Western style diet, such as consumption of fruit juices, carbonated soft- and other lifestyle-drinks; while the children from a background with a lower-education level continued the use of traditional drinks. In contrast to these findings, Harding et al. [33] found a relationship between low socioeconomic status, frequent consumption of fruit squash and carbonated drinks and the occurrence of dental erosion. In this study, it was not assessed if the children from the low socioeconomic background had more plaque, which would be a diffusion barrier for erosion.

Intrinsic Factor

Gastroesophageal Reflux and Vomiting
It is well known, that newborn babies often have gastroesophageal reflux (GOR) which decreases over the first year of life. After the age of one, 8% of the children continue to suffer from GOR [34]. This condition seems to be an important etiological factor for dental erosion in children [35, 36]. In another study, the prevalence of dental erosion in children with GOR, aged between 2 and 16 years, was low compared to a regular population. The authors suggested that in children refluxing is often limited to the esophagus and therefore no erosive lesions of the teeth are generated. It was concluded that dental

erosion might not be as great a problem in children with GOR disease as it is in adults [37].

More studies investigating the impact of regurgitation and vomiting on the teeth are discussed in chapter 8. It is important to remember, in daily clinical practice that children often will not report reflux because, for them, it is silent or regarded as normal.

Case Report

Patient M.R., Male, 8 Years

Case History
The patient was sent to the clinic by the dentist because of advanced erosive tooth wear found on the deciduous teeth and slight wear found on the permanent teeth. In general, the boy was healthy but he suffered from dentine hypersensitivity, especially in the right maxillary area. His parents reported that their child vomited regularly until the age of 1½ years. The patient himself said that each morning he has slime present in his mouth. At presentation, he was still vomiting approximately 6 times per year. Nutritional case history taking (the patient had to note each nutrition intake for four consecutive days including a weekend) showed no pathology; on average, the boy had two acid inputs per day, which is considered below the threshold of the critical value of four acid inputs per day.

Clinical Findings
Clinical examination showed multiple oral and occlusal erosion lesions. The deciduous molars had advanced erosive defects with dentinal involvement. The first permanent molars and the lingual surfaces of the upper permanent incisors showed erosive tooth wear confined to enamel (figs. 1, 3, 4). The facial tooth surfaces were seldom involved and only slight defects were found. The examination of the saliva parameters showed no pathological values. Flow rate of resting saliva was 0.8 ml/min; buffering capacity was low to regular as measured with a commercially available indicator system (Dentobuff, Vivadent, Schaan, Liechtenstein). The pH of saliva was 7.1. However, the pH of the slime collected after sleeping in the morning was 5.0 (Merck, Darmstadt, Germany).

Because of the localization of the erosive defects and the clinical findings, an intrinsic cause was presumed and the patient was referred to a gastroenterologist. In parallel, preventive measures were started.

Preventive Measures
To stop or at least to reduce the erosive process a topical fluoride varnish was applied on the erosive defects (Duraphat, Colgate-Palmolive, Thalwil, Switzerland). In addition, the patient was instructed to rinse with a fluoride mouth-rinse, twice a day (Meridol, Gaba AG, Therwil, Switzerland). In order to reduce dentine hypersensitivity; a sealer was applied to the hypersensitive areas (Seal and Protect, Dentsply de Trey, Konstanz, Germany) and the patient was advised to gently apply a topical fluoride gel twice a week (Elmex gel, Gaba AG, Therwil, Switzerland) (fig. 2).

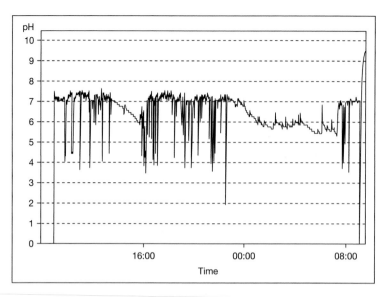

Fig. 5. 24-Hour pH measurements in the esophagus of the boy after a 2-year period of medication with omeprazol. A strong reduction of the GOR is apparent. pH was below 4 for only 3% of the measurement time.

Initial Clinical Diagnosis and Outcome

The patient refused the gastroenterological examination with pH telemetry, however he was possibly too young to understand and consent for this treatment. The erosive tooth wear progressed in spite of the preventive measures. Therefore, at the age of 11.5 years the patient agreed to a second attempt to an esophago-gastro-duodenoscopy with no pathological findings detected. Further to this, a 24-h pH measurement was made. This found the pH in the distal esophagus to be below 5.5 for 10 h and below pH 4 for more than 4% of the measurement time. These values are regarded as pathological. The episodes of GOR occurred overnight while sleeping or directly after ingestion of food or drink.

Based on the gastroenterological and dental investigations, a diagnosis was made of dental erosion caused by GOR.

Therapy

To reduce the secretion of gastric acid an omeprazol medicament was prescribed (Antramups, Astra Zeneca, 2 times per day 20 mg). The patient was advised to continue with the application of fluoride to the teeth and to not sleep in a flat, horizontal position, to prevent refluxing.

Further Clinical Investigation and Treatment

A further 24 h pH investigation at the age of 13 years showed a strong reduction in the GOR (fig. 5). It was concluded that, as a part of the physiological growth, the sphincter of the

---

Lussi/Jaeggi

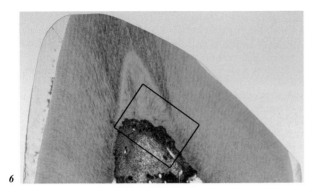

6

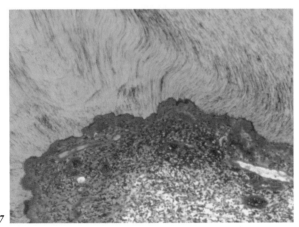

7

Figs. 6, 7. Histological section of a deciduous canine after exfoliation: Denuded primary dentine and reactionary dentine with intact dentinal tubules are present explaining the hypersensitivity the patient suffered from (same patient as in figs. 1–5).

esophagus worked more effectively. Based on the decreased reflux values, the medicament therapy was ceased.

No further progression of erosive tooth wear was observed, which prevented the need for invasive restorative therapy of the erosive defects by means of composite fillings, veneers or crowns.

This case clearly demonstrates that a conservative approach to treatment, such as fluoride therapy and sealing of hypersensitive dentine to prevent further tooth erosion, is the first choice, as long as no progression of the condition is observed.

After exfoliation of the deciduous teeth, the patient put them at our disposal, which allowed histological examination to be performed. Figures 6 and 7 show the histological sections of a primary canine with advanced erosion extending into dentine. Due to a relatively moderate irritation the primary odontoblasts survived and were able to produce reactionary dentine. The formation of this can be explained by the clinical findings of dentine hypersensitivity, as a communication between the denuded surface of the dentinal tubules and the pulp was present.

References

1   Millward A, Shaw L, Smith AJ: Dental erosion in four-year-old children from differing socio-economic backgrounds. ASDC J Dent Child 1994;61:263–266.
2   Jones SG, Nunn JH: The dental health of 3-year-old children in east Cumbria 1993. Community Dent Health 1995;12:161–166.
3   Hunter ML, West NX, Hughes JA, Newcombe RG, Addy M: Erosion of deciduous and permanent dental hard tissue in the oral environment. J Dent 2000;28:257–263.
4   Amaechi BT, Higham SM, Edgar WM: Factors influencing the development of dental erosion in vitro: enamel type, temperature and exposure time. J Oral Rehabil 1999;26:624–630.
5   Hunter ML, West NX, Hughes JA, Newcombe RG, Addy M: Relative susceptibility of deciduous and permanent dental hard tissues to erosion by a low pH fruit drink in vitro. J Dent 2000;28: 265–270.
6   Maupomé G, Aguilar-Avila M, Medrano-Ugalde H, Borges-Yanez A: In vitro quantitative micro-hardness assessment of enamel with early salivary pellicles after exposure to an eroding cola drink. Caries Res 1999;33:140–147.
7   Lussi A, Kohler N, Zero D, Schaffner M, Megert B: A comparison of the erosive potential of different beverages in primary and permanent teeth using an in vitro model. Eur J Oral Sci 2000;108:110–114.
8   Lussi A, Schaffner M, Jaeggi T, Grüninger A: Erosionen: Befund – Diagnose – Risikofaktoren – Prävention – Therapie. Schweiz Monatsschr Zahnmed 2005:115:917–935.
9   Lippert F, Parker DM, Jandt KD: Susceptibility of deciduous and permanent enamel to dietary acid-induced erosion studied with atomic force microscopy nanoindentation. Eur J Oral Sci 2004;112:61–66.
10 Johansson AK, Sorvari R, Birkhed D, Meurman JH: Dental erosion in deciduous teeth – an in vivo and in vitro study. J Dent 2001;29:333–340.
11 Attin T, Koidl U, Buchalla W, Schaller HG, Kielbassa AM, Hellwig E: Correlation of microhard-ness and wear in differently eroded bovine dental enamel. Arch Oral Biol 1997;42:243–250.
12 Milosevic A, Lennon MA, Fear SC: Risk factors associated with tooth wear in teenagers: a case control study. Community Dent Health 1997;14:143–147.
13 Järvinen VK, Rytomaa II, Heinonen OP: Risk factors in dental erosion. J Dent Res 1991;70: 942–947.
14 Lussi A, Jaeggi T, Zero D: The role of diet in the aetiology of dental erosion. Caries Res 2004;38: 34–44.
15 Dugmore CR, Rock WP: A multifactorial analysis of factors associated with dental erosion. Br Dent J 2004;196:283–286.
16 Unesda-Cisda: Total consumption of non-alcoholic beverages in Europe 2003. www.unesda-cisda.org
17 Rugg-Gunn AJ, Lennon MA, Brown JG: Sugar consumption in the United Kingdom. Br Dent J 1987;167:339–364.
18 Gleason P, Suitor C: Children's Diets in the Mid-1990s: Dietary Intake and Its Relationship with School Meal Participation. Alexandria, US Department of Agriculture, Food and Nutrition Service, Office of Analysis, Nutrition and Evaluation, 2001.
19 American Academy of Pediatrics, Committee on School Health: Soft drinks in schools. Pediatrics 2004;113:152–153.
20 Al-Dlaigan YH, Shaw L, Smith AJ: Dental erosion in a group of British 14-year-old school chil-dren. II. Influence of dietary intake. Br Dent J 2001;190:258–261.
21 Sanchez GA, Fernandez De Preliasco MV: Salivary pH changes during soft drinks consumption in children. Int J Paediatr Dent 2003;13:251–257.
22 Smith AJ, Shaw L: Baby fruits juices and tooth erosion. Br Dent J 1987;162:65–67.
23 Luo Y, Zeng XJ, Du MQ, Bedi R: The prevalence of dental erosion in preschool children in China. J Dent 2005;33:115–121.
24 Nunn JH, Gordon PH, Morris AJ, Pine CM, Walker A: Dental erosion – changing prevalence? A review of British National childrens' surveys. Int J Paediatr Dent 2003;13:98–105.

25 Al-Dlaigan YH, Shaw L, Smith AJ: Vegetarian children and dental erosion. Int J Paediatr Dent 2001;11:184–192.
26 Sullivan RE, Kramer WS: Iatrogenic erosion of teeth. J Dent Child 1983;50:192–196.
27 Asher C, Read MJF: Early enamel erosion in children associated with the excessive consumption of citric acid. Br Dent J 1987;162:384–387.
28 Al-Dlaigan YH, Shaw L, Smith AJ: Is there a relationship between asthma and dental erosion? A case control study. Int J Paediatr Dent 2002;12:189–200.
29 Shaw L, Al-Dlaigan YH, Smith AJ: Childhood asthma and dental erosion. ASDC J Dent Child 2000;67:102–106.
30 Dugmore CR, Rock WP: Asthma and tooth erosion. Is there an association? Int J Paediatr Dent 2003;13:417–424.
31 O'Sullivan EA, Curzon ME: A comparison of acidic dietary factors in children with and without dental erosion. ASDC J Dent Child 2000;67:186–192.
32 O'Sullivan EA, Curzon ME: Dental erosion associated with the use of 'alcopop': a case report. Br Dent J 1998;184:594–596.
33 Harding MA, Whelton H, O'Mullane DM, Cronin M: Dental erosion in 5-year-old Irish school children and associated factors: a pilot study. Community Dental Health 2003;20:165–170.
34 Osatakul S, Sriplung H, Puetpaiboon A, Junjana CO, Chamnongpakdi S: Prevalence and natural course of gastroesophageal reflux symptoms: a 1-year cohort study in Thai infants. J Pediatr Gastroenterol Nutr 2002;34:63–67.
35 Linnet V, Seow WK: Dental erosion in children: a literature review. Pediatr Dent 2001;23:37–43.
36 Dahshan A, Patel H, Delaney J, Wuerth A, Thomas R, Tolia V: Gastroesophageal reflux disease and dental erosion in children. J Pediatr 2002;140:474–478.
37 O'Sullivan EA, Curzon ME, Roberts GJ, Milla PJ, Stringer MD: Gastroesophageal reflux in children and its relationship to erosion of primary and permanent teeth. Eur J Oral Sci 1998;106:765–769.

Prof. Dr. Adrian Lussi
Department of Preventive, Restorative and Pediatric Dentistry
School of Dental Medicine
University of Bern
Freiburgstrasse 7
CH–3010 Bern (Switzerland)

Lussi A (ed): Dental Erosion.
Monogr Oral Sci. Basel, Karger, 2006, vol 20, pp 152–172

·····················

Methods for Assessment of Dental Erosion

Thomas Attin

Center for Dental and Oral Medicine and Maxillo-facial Surgery,
Clinic for Preventive Dentistry, Periodontology and Cariology,
University of Zurich, Zürich, Switzerland

Abstract

Various assessment techniques have been applied to evaluate the loss of dental hard tissue and the surface-softened zone in enamel induced by erosive challenges. In this chapter, the most frequently adopted techniques for analyzing the erosively altered dental hard tissues are reviewed, such as profilometry, microradiography, scanning electron microscopy, atom force microscopy, nano- and microhardness tests and iodide permeability test. Moreover, methods for chemical analysis of minerals dissolved from dental hard tissue are discussed. It becomes evident that the complex nature of erosive mineral loss and dissolution might not be comprehended by a single technique, but needs application of different approaches for full understanding.

Acid attack leads to an irreversible loss of the outermost enamel and dentin layers and to partial demineralization (softening) of the tooth surface. In enamel, the thickness of the softened layer is estimated to be 2–5 μm [1, 2]. The softened eroded tooth surface is highly susceptible to abrasive wear, and mechanical impacts such as toothbrushing can easily remove the superficially demineralized dental hard tissue [3–5].

For simulating intra-oral erosion as closely as possible, it is desirable to assess the erosive effects on native tooth surfaces. Most of the methods described below need polished surfaces for precise assessment of the erosively induced defects or for creating reference surfaces, which means that the natural, often fluoridated surface of the tooth has to be removed. However, it should be considered that in the case of intra-oral erosion the outermost surface layers are also continuously removed by the acid attack, so that a 'polished' surface is created. When monitoring of erosive surface alterations within a period of time is performed, it could become necessary to fix a specimen in the measuring device in a reproducible position. This aspect becomes increasingly more important the smaller the mineral loss is.

In the oral cavity, the contact of the teeth with an acidic substrate is usually limited to a few seconds before clearance by saliva. This means that under natural conditions an early erosive lesion is created with very small loss of mineral and erosive craters in a nanometer scale or even a near-atomic level. Detection of these small surface changes would allow reducing the contact of an acidic substrate with the tooth surface in experiments to a time period resembling intra-oral conditions. Moreover, feasibility to detect these small alterations would enable one to reduce contact of the substrate with a tooth to a single and short event instead of long or repeated procedures which are disadvantageous in in situ and in vitro experiments. When erosion is assessed in dentin specimens, it is important to notice that drying of a dentin may lead to shrinkage of the specimen rendering the detection of small surface alterations and loss difficult.

It has, however, to be noted that assessment procedures should fulfill intra-assay (coefficient of variation of <10%) and inter-assay precision with time (coefficient of variation of <20%) according to the guidance for bioanalytical methods as recently described [6, 7]. Moreover, lower limits of quantification should be determined before application of a method meaning that only those readings should be considered in the analysis that are higher than the value of detection limit plus 5 × SD [6, 7]. The limit of detection and the precision of a method may depend on the substrate to be analyzed, so that these parameters could not be taken from manufacturers' descriptions, since recently exemplarily shown for a calcium assay [8]. Unfortunately, only in few erosion studies are these parameters clearly given for the specific assessment methods applied. Generally, qualitative assessments bear the problem that classification and interpretation of the findings is more or less subjective depending on the investigator. In order to get objective and measurable data, quantitative analyses should be preferred when possible. However, with qualitative determinations [such as SEM and confocal laser scanning microscopy (CLSM)] changes of tooth structure could be visualized giving an impression to the reader of the different impacts of different substrates on the dental hard tissues.

Due to the lack of fixed intra-oral reference points, it is complicated to monitor the progression of erosive tooth wear accurately on natural tooth surfaces in the oral cavity. Moreover, most of the devices used for detection of mineral loss and changes could only be performed on especially prepared specimens. Therefore, erosive and erosive/abrasive alterations of dental hard tissues are mostly investigated either in in vitro studies or in in situ studies. In the latter ones, enamel or dentin specimens are extra-orally or sometimes intra-orally subjected to erosive challenges, worn in the oral cavity according to the intra-oral cariogenicity test developed by [9–11] and finally assessed in the laboratory for hard tissue loss and surface alterations.

Due to the two patterns – loss and softening of the dental hard tissue – assessments of dental erosions deal with different methodological approaches, namely to evaluate either surface phenomena only, such as change of surface hardness, or the loss of the dental hard tissues per se. Various techniques have been used to investigate these two aspects of dental erosion [12, 13].

In the following, the most established and well-evaluated techniques as well as emerging methods will be described.

Scanning Electron Microscopy

With scanning electron microscopy (SEM) surface alterations after erosive attacks are qualitatively estimated. Grading of the severity of surface alteration could be done on individually adopted scales. SEM investigations can be performed on both polished and unpolished, native surfaces after gold-sputtering. In enamel, acid attacks due to immersion of specimens in erosive solutions lead to a surface etching pattern with exposition of enamel prisms to an extent depending on the severity of the erosive challenge. SEM investigations were also applied for evaluating the efficacy of salivary acquired pellicle to protect underlying enamel surface from acidic dissolution [14–16] or to demonstrate superficially deposited precipitates resulting from mineral dissolution with differently acting acids [17]. In dentin, acid treatments may result in opening of the dentin tubules which could be graded according to its degree [18]. With common scanning electron microscopes, moisture loss of specimens due to necessary preparation of the specimens for the SEM investigation may lead to additional alterations of the eroded surface. To avoid collapse of the fragile eroded enamel surface structure, freeze drying of samples was suggested [19]. Precipitates formed by dissolved enamel mineral may block the enamel surface so that the eroded enamel prism structure might not be seen with SEM. To reduce the risk of artefactual reprecipitation, neutralization of the acid is recommended before removal of samples from the acidic bath. Impregnation of the delicate surface with methacrylate or dentin adhesives allows for fabrication of resin replicas [20]. After complete dissolution of the enamel with HCl, the resin replicas could then be studied with SEM providing insight into structural surface and subsurface changes.

With environmental SEM (ESEM), no sample preparation is required, reducing the risk for artefacts to a minimum. ESEM also allows for examination of samples without metal or carbon coating, respectively, in low vacuum and in wet conditions. Nevertheless, SEM and ESEM technique does not provide as detailed information about surface alterations of eroded samples as other methods used for the evaluation of erosive impact on dental hard tissues.

SEM or ESEM could be coupled with energy dispersive X-ray spectroscopy and was also used for a microanalysis suitable for analyzing elemental distribution in the top few micrometers of a sample surface. An electron beam hitting the surface leads to excitement of atoms resulting in emitting of X-rays which may provide information about distribution of various elements, such as calcium, phosphate and carbon with a concentration of about 1 wt%. However, suitability of the method for evaluating erosive processes has not been clearly demonstrated as yet [21].

Both SEM and ESEM are suitable for use with native surfaces. Although, both methods do only allow subjective, qualitative assessment. ESEM is favorable when wet substrates or dentin should be evaluated.

Surface Hardness Measurements

For determining changes of surface hardness of erosively altered dental hard tissues, microhardness and, as a relatively new approach, nanoindentation techniques are often used. With hardness measurements, early stages of enamel and dentin dissolution, which are associated with weakening of the surface, can be determined. The basic method of micro- and nanoindentation involves the indentation of a diamond tip of known geometrical dimensions for a given load and duration.

For microhardness assessments of eroded tooth surfaces, mostly the diamonds according to Knoop or Vickers used on previously polished surfaces. Polished surfaces are recommended to produce well-defined indentations. Application of Knoop diamond resulted in a rhomboid indentation, Vickers in a tetra-pyramidal one. The lengths of the indentations on the surface are measured under a microscope requiring indentations lengths of about 30–40 μm length for precise measurements. By means of a special formula Knoop or Vickers hardness numbers are calculated. In enamel, length of the indentations is not time-dependent and could be recorded immediately. However, in dentin, indentation length changed due to flexibility of the dentin substrate, which was shown for indentations performed with 500 g. In this case, indentations should best be measured 24 h after having made the indentation [22]. No comparable recommendations are available for dentin indentations conducted with lower forces, although it could be assumed that when applying low forces the time needed to retraction of dentin after loading might be shorter than 24 h. On erosively altered surfaces, the outlines of the indentations are sometimes fuzzy rendering precise measurements difficult. The hardness measured by indentation is affected not only by the immediate surrounding, but also by changes of the material in a distance of approximately 10 times the dimensions of the indentation. To limit the impact of surrounding material changes, microindentations for determining erosive alterations of the superficial surfaces are performed with low pressure of about 50 g (0.49 N) [23, 24]. Nevertheless, one should be aware that microhardness measurements do not reflect the properties of the surface only. The penetration depth of the Vickers diamond amounted to 1/7 of indentation length; i.e. with indentations from, e.g., 35 µm length, the depth of penetration amounts to 5.0 µm. Penetration depth of the Knoop diamond amounts to 1/30.5 of its indentation length. This means that with same indentation length and visibility under the assessment microscope the Knoop hardness determination better reflects alterations of the actually outermost layers than the Vickers hardness testing, since Knoop hardness indentations from, e.g., 35 µm length are equivalent to a penetration depth of 1.15 µm. Nevertheless, microhardness measurements such as the Knoop procedure allow discriminating different erosive potentials of various substances on dental hard tissue, even after short exposures (3 min) to acidic agents [25]. In other studies, immersion periods of at least 20 min were chosen to investigate the impact on surface hardness [23, 26, 27].

By means of the indentations on enamel surfaces detection of enamel abrasion is also possible by calculating the depth of the indentations. The difference between the depth before and the depth after abrasion provided a direct measurement for the loss of substance by abrasion at this site [28, 29]. The main principle behind this method is that the body of the indentation is not changed and not removed by the abrasion. Only the surrounding tissue on the surface is removed so that due to the pyramidal geometry the contour of the indentation (an thereby its length) is reduced [28, 29]. The substance loss (Δd) is calculated from the change in indentation length (Δl) using the geometrical formula: $\Delta d = 0.032772 \, \Delta l$. With this procedure, surface loss due to abrasion of previously eroded samples of about 30–100 nm could be determined precisely [30, 31]. Unfortunately, measurements of the amount of substance directly removed by an erosive attack could not be performed with this method, since the acid also removes some substance from the body of the indentation and not only from its surrounding.

In another approach, Schweizer-Hirt et al. [32] visually compared different degrees of disappearance of the indentations after enamel erosion–abrasion, thus estimating substance loss.

The main advantages of microhardness determinations are the relatively low costs, the long experience with the system and the fact that it could be combined with measurements of abrasive surface loss.

Surface Profilometry

Using a surface profilometer (surfometer) irreversible loss of dental hard tissue and surface roughness could be determined by scanning specimens with a laser beam or a contact stylus (metal or diamond) with a diameter of about 2–20 μm [4, 33–36]. The contact stylus is loaded with a force of a few milli-Newtons. With the scan, a complete map of the specimen surface could be generated. However, the outermost demineralized layer of enamel erosions is very damageable to mechanical forces so that profilometer measurements will be effected by the tendency of the stylus to penetrate this fragile layer.

Application of the laser beam leads to higher resolution as compared to the contact stylus (resolution on accuracy in height ~10 nm). However, the laser stylus may produce 'overshots' at the sharp edges at the bottom of grooves which result in artefacts [37]. It should also be noted that dissolution of the enamel due to acid attack leads to surface roughening of about 0.4 μm. Therefore, reliable detection of minimal losses below 1 μm are generally difficult to accomplish with profilometry, although Hooper et al. [38] have demonstrated that profilometry was able to distinguish between different abrasivities of toothpastes creating hard tissue loss of about 0.5 μm. For such precise measurements with low variations, meticulous flattening and polishing of sample surface is an important step.

In studies using surfometry, parts of the surface are protected by nail varnish or adhesive tape prior to the erosive or abrasive attack to produce reference areas allowing comparison between the levels of the untreated and treated surfaces. However, it is also possible to match the baseline scan recorded with the scan conducted after treatment in a computer in order to determine differences in height between these two scans with a special software [39, 40]. In this case, it is extremely important to ensure correct repositioning of the sample in the profilometer for the two readings.

Commonly, polished surfaces are used in profilometry studies, since native enamel or dentin surface show an intrinsic coarseness rendering detection of small changes due to erosion/abrasion impossible. However, in natural enamel extended depths of at least 50 μm of erosive grooves could also be measured without the need for preparation (polishing) of the surface [34].

Chadwick et al. [41] presented a method to obtain digital surface models using electroconductive replicas generated from silicone impressions of teeth taken at different time points. The replicas were used for surface mapping, by means of a computer-controlled probe. Resolution in z-direction is reported to be 1 μm [42]. The resultant maps may be compared using a surface matching and difference detection algorithm. This technique provides readings with good accuracy and reproducibility [43–45]. Erosions of 50 μm magnitude occurring over a 9 month period were recorded to a precision of about ±15 μm [42].

As summarized, profilometry is a method, which may be adopted for surface loss with high precision provided that material loss exceeds about 0.4 μm. The method is also applicable for indirect measurements of intra-oral erosions via replicas.

Iodide Permeability Test

Iodide permeability tests (IPT) were introduced by Bakhos et al. [46] and is based on the principle that defined areas of enamel samples are allowed to soak for a few minutes with potassium iodide which is recovered from the enamel by Millipore prefilter paper discs. The amount of iodide recovered in the discs is determined and provides information about the pore volume of the enamel. It was shown that (IPT) measurements are closely related to the pore volume of enamel and give sensitive estimations of the early stages of de- and remineralization [47]. Moreover, it was proven that a linear relationship between IP and calcium loss exists [48]. Changes of enamel structure recorded with IPT have also been shown to correlate well with microhardness testing. This was true for severely eroded samples, in which erosions were performed by immersion in lactate (pH 4.75) for a minimum of 60 min [49]. With shorter exposure periods in the erosive solution, the two methods did not correlate well in this study. Lussi et al. [26] showed that exposure to acidic drinks leads to an increase in IP which was significantly associated with the acidity, pH, and mineral contents of the drinks. In contrast to the aforementioned study, Lussi et al. [26] found a correlation between IP and microhardness data for enamel samples immersed in acidic beverages for a period of 20 min.

The IP method has the advantage that low costs are involved with this approach, which allows more or less rapid screening of the impact of different erosive substances on enamel.

Chemical Analysis of Minerals Dissolved in the Erosive Agent

Dental enamel consists of 34–39% m/m (g per 100 g) calcium (dry weight) and 16–18% m/m phosphorus [50]. Therefore, determination of dental enamel dissolution by assessing the amount of calcium or phosphate dissolved from the apatite crystals of dental hard tissue could also be regarded as a possible tool for assessing dental erosions. Hence, some authors had applied calcium determination in erosive, acidic solutions after prolonged contact (range 2 min to 24 h) of the solutions with dental hard tissue using calcium sensitive electrodes or atomic adsorption spectrophotometer [51–55]. Calcium-sensitive electrodes often need a specific pH of the environment to work precisely. Additionally, calcium complexes formed with certain acids (e.g. citric acid) impair correct measurements of the calcium released from the dental hard tissue. Atomic absorption spectrophotometer requires intensive preparation of the solution to allow for measurement of calcium or phosphate. Both methods additionally need solution volumes exceeding a minimum of $100\,\mu l$. Atomic absorption spectrophotometer uses the adsorption of light, usually from a hollow-cathode lamp of the element that is being measured, to determine the concentration of gas-phase atoms. Since samples are usually liquids or solids, the analyte atoms or ions must be vaporized in a flame or graphite furnace. The atoms absorb ultraviolet or visible light and make transitions to higher electronic energy levels. The analyte concentration is determined from the amount of absorption. Concentration measurements are usually determined from a working curve after calibrating the instrument with standards of known concentration. Recently, the colorimetric Arsenazo III method was described allowing precise determination in acidic solution of small volumes of $10\,\mu l$ in a spectrophotometer [8, 17]. However, this method also could not be applied in all kind of acids with the same precision. In colorimetric methods, absorbance of light due to the formed colored complex is related to the quantity of the analyte. It should be noted that formation of the colored complex might be impaired by other agents in the solution or by pH.

Determination of phosphorus released during the dissolution process is mostly performed by colorimetric methods such as the ammonium-(phospho-) molybdate method [56, 57]. Another colorimetric method, with a 10 times higher sensitivity, is the phosphomolybdate-malachite green procedure [58] which has shown to be suitable for determination of phosphate dissolved from enamel after etching with perchloric acid at a range of $0.025–3.0\,mM$ [59]. Recent studies corroborated this fact showing that, depending on the acid used, the malachite green procedure is a reliable and suitable tool to detect and quantify minimal phosphate contents in small samples of a variety of acidic solutions which have the potential to form erosive lesions [60].

The chemical methods for assessment of erosive dissolution have the advantage that they allow detection of very small mineral loss using unpolished, native tooth samples. As yet, these methods were only applied in in vitro experiments.

Microradiography

Microradiography is a tool for quantification of mineral loss based on the attenuation of X-ray irradiation transmitting dental hard tissue. X-ray photons transmitting a dental hard tissue sample can be recorded by photo-counting X-ray detectors, or X-ray sensitive photographic plates or film. The mineral mass can be calculated from the photon counts or gray values of photographic plates or film knowing the appropriate mass attenuation coefficient or by determining photographic density measurements calibrated by an aluminum step-wedge [61–63]. For gray value assessment of photographic plates or film densitometers or, more recently, CCD cameras attached to a microscope are in use.

Microradiography has been frequently used in studies determining mineral changes due to de- and remineralization in terms of caries. The method was used for studying these processes in early enamel lesions and less frequently in dentin. For transverse microradiography (TMR) thin sections (50–200 μm) are obtained perpendicular to the sample surface and radiographed with a Nickel-filtered Cu Kα-line (i.e. at 20 kV, 20 mA) perpendicular to the cut surface. Due to limitations in specimen preparation and alignment, and the geometry of the X-ray beam that spreads radial from a point or line focus rather than parallel, the imaging precision at the sample edge is limited. Usually, the outermost 5–10 μm cannot be exactly reproduced. In early enamel caries with the typical subsurface lesion, mineral loss and changes predominantly occur in the body of the lesion below the pseudo-intact surface layer at about 20–50 μm thickness and beyond [64]. TMR is a valid tool for quantitative assessment of the mineral content as a function of depth from the surface of caries and caries-like lesions. From in-depth profiles, the lesion depth and mineral loss integrated over the entire depth (IML or ΔZ) of the lesion can be calculated. Lesion depth usually is defined up to that point, where the mineral content reaches 95% of the mineral content of sound enamel or dentin.

Beyond its original use in caries research, microradiography was adopted for detecting erosive mineral loss. In a TMR-like setup thin enamel or dentin sections can be used to measure erosive mineral loss. In this case, the erosive agent is applied on the cut surface that also contains reference areas not subjected to erosion and X-ray images are taken [65]. Note that in contrast to TMR, as is usually applied in caries research, the erosion is performed on the cut surface of an already prepared tooth slice of 100–200 μm thickness rather than on a specimen's surface that is cut perpendicularly for TMR after an experimental procedure. Hall et al. [65] found a strong correlation between mineral loss determined by either TMR or profilometry even for discrimination of early erosive lesions caused by erosion times of less than 1 h.

Another approach to use TMR for erosive mineral loss determination also depends on the use of reference areas not subjected to an erosive challenge [66]. The erosive challenge is executed on a specimens' surface. Then a slice (50–200 μm) is prepared perpendicular to the surface the same way as for traditional TMR. Thereby, both depth of the erosive crater and the depth below the

Attin

bottom of the crater at which mineral content was reduced (surface softening) can be assessed with TMR giving lesion depth and integrated mineral loss as variables [67, 68]. In these studies, TMR was used to record lesion depths from 20 μm and more. For determination of mineral changes following a small erosive challenge, e.g. erosive surface softening only, this technique is not sensitive enough due to the fuzziness of the outer 5–10 μm at the edge of the dental hard tissue slabs prepared for TMR.

Longitudinal microradiography (LMR) enables the use of thicker specimens up to 4 mm thickness usually cut from the tooth comprising the natural enamel surface and some underlying dentin. However, use of thinner specimens provides better information about the mineral change within the specimen. The specimens are radiographed perpendicular to the surface before (reference) and after treatment(s), and changes in mineral content can be calculated using pixel by pixel comparison of gray values of a radiograph after treatment with the gray values of the reference radiograph. In contrast to TMR, LMR is not able to determine the mineral profile of a specimen from the surface to depth. Since LMR enables the reuse of specimens, it can be used for longitudinal observations. The mineral loss recorded with LMR consists of both the erosive crater and the loss of mineral in the softened surface zone. LMR is less sensitive to minute changes in mineral content than TMR, because of the use of thicker specimens as compared with TMR.

Using LMR, erosion progression in both enamel and dentin has also been assessed [69–71]. In these studies, the method has shown to be suitable to allow for distinction of different preventive treatment modalities resulting in different mineral loss. A recently published comparison of LMR in enamel specimens with either profilometry or analysis of dissolved calcium/phosphorus showed good correlation for the three methods [72]. However, it also became clear that losses below 20 μm should be interpreted with care when using LMR only, since standard deviations were quite high when determining minimal substance loss with LMR.

The main advantage of microradiography is that the method enables to simultaneously determine surface loss and demineralization of the eroded samples.

Confocal Laser Scanning Microscopy

CLSM is a tool for obtaining high-resolution images, 3-D reconstructions and optical sections through 3-D specimens. The translucency of teeth allows nondestructive subsurface visualization of their microstructure by CLSM used in reflection mode at a level of about 150–200 μm below the surface [73–75]. Although mostly polished tooth samples are used for CLSM, also unpolished and even wet tooth substrates could be assessed with the method. However, quality of images obtained from unpolished samples is limited due to reflections and scattering effects caused by the uneven surface. Moreover, surfaces of polished samples could quite easily be aligned parallel to the ground which is required to obtain images from a defined subsurface level.

In brief, CLSM works as follows: illumination, provided by a gas laser (e.g. Ar/Kr or He/Ar) is focused by an objective lens into a small focal volume within a fluorescent specimen. The laser beam, which could be filtered to select specific wavelengths (often 488 nm) is thereby focused on the focal plane. A mixture of emitted fluorescent light as well as reflected laser light from the illuminated spot is then recollected by the objective lenses and a photon multiplier detector. The focus plane of illumination is the same as the focal plane of detection, which means that they are confocal. Information of the specimen can be collected from different focal planes by raising or lowering the microscopes stage. The computer can generate a 3-D picture of a sample by assembling a stack of these 2-D images from successive focal planes.

Used in erosion studies, CLSM provides histotomographic images allowing for qualitative assessment and interpretation of hard tissue destruction or mineral dissolution, since light reflection and light scattering of hard tissue samples are influenced by micro-histological changes within a tooth sample [76–78]. Since these images provide only limited information about the exact degree of demineralization, CLSM is mostly combined with other methods (e.g. microhardness, analysis of mineral loss or others).

The main advantage of CLSM is the high resolution of the system providing a 3-D insight into the erosively altered substrate.

Quantitative Light-Induced Fluorescence

Quantitative light-induced fluorescence (QLF) was developed as a nondestructive diagnostic method for the longitudinal assessment of early caries lesions [79]. The method applies a xenon gas discharge lamp to illuminate a tooth with filtered blue–violet light to provoke its natural fluorescence. The natural fluorescence is assumed to be caused by fluorophores, which are predominately located at the dentin–enamel junction and in dentin. Due to higher scattering in carious enamel less excitation light reaches the fluorescing dentin–enamel junction and underlying dentin and less fluorescence from the dentin–enamel junction and dentin is able to find its way back through the carious lesion. Therefore, the lesion appears dark in contrast to the surrounding, fluorescing area of the tooth. The area of interest is imaged by a CCD video camera through an optical high-pass filter that blocks the excitation light and allows only the fluorescing light to pass. The averaged difference in fluorescence intensity (ΔF [%]) between the darker fluorescing lesion area and the brighter fluorescing sound area around the lesion is calculated by proprietary software.

As yet, QLF was applied in two studies for monitoring erosive lesions [80, 81]. The method was validated in comparison to TMR and was found to be an effective tool for quantification of erosive defects. As already mentioned, the erosive lesion comprises a crater and a softened demineralized surface layer. It could be assumed that the softened surface layer is too thin to create scattering effects of light to such an extent as observed in carious lesions, so that the demineralized surface layer could not account for the loss of fluorescence of the erosive lesion. Therefore, it was hypothesized that the walls of the crater of the erosion are primarily responsible for the dark appearance of the lesion when assessed with QLF. It was assumed that the walls create a shadowing effect and that they hinder release of the fluorescing light due to scattering. With an increase of the depth of the crater, these effects might also increase leading to a more pronounced accentuation of the erosive defect when assessed with QLF. However, the principle behind the reduced fluorescence of erosive lesions is not fully understood and needs to be clarified in further experiments.

Atomic Force Microscopy

Atomic force microscopes (AFM) as well as scanning tunneling microscopes are pertaining to the family of scanning probe microscopes. In the following, some properties of the instrument are given as already described in detail elsewhere [13, 21, 82]. The main application of AFM is high resolution imaging of different materials including polymers, ceramics, metals, biomolecules and cells. Different operation modes allow measurement of among others surface topography, lateral surface composition and differences in elasticity. Ultra-sharp probes with radii of 4–60 nm are connected to a flexible cantilever and accurate ceramic piezo-elements, which allow the sample to be scanned with sub-nanometer precision. The cantilever deflects in the z-direction due to the surface topography during tip scanning over the surface. A diode laser beam is reflected from the back of the cantilever and is incident on a four-segment photodiode. As the tip moves, the deflection of the cantilever is indicated by the position of the laser on the photodiode, thus constructing a map of the sample surface [21]. The tip can move over the sample in dynamic modes with an oscillating tip moving up and down in either tapping mode (with touching surface contacts) or noncontact mode. In noncontact modes, the tip is placed at the level of the attractive van der Waals forces to detect force gradients. In nondynamic modes, the tip is moved laterally in constant contact with the surface (contact mode). AFM can be used equally well on conducting and insulating materials in ambient conditions, in air or liquids. The resolution is orders of magnitude greater than with profilometry, however, scan size is limited to at most $0.5 \times 0.5\,mm^2$ taking some 60 min for this size.

AFM was used in erosion studies for qualitative approaches comparing the surface of dental hard tissue and acquired enamel pellicle after exposure to different erosive agents [83–85]. Moreover, substance loss of enamel due to erosion was determined with tapping mode [84] with high resolution. Generally, AFM is able to measure height differences in the order of the size of one atom rendering the technique suitable for detection of very early stages of substance loss due to erosive and abrasive attacks.

Nanoindentation

For nanoindentation, an indenter diamond is applied on dental hard tissue with small loads in the order of nN to mN. Therefore, the indentation depth of the indenter tip could be limited to about 100 nm allowing for measurements in the outermost softened layer. Mostly, a Berkovich diamond tip is used resulting in a three-sided pyramidal indentation. The indenter is driven into the sample by applying increasing load to some preset value. The load is gradually decreased until partial or complete relaxation of the sample has occurred. The load and displacement are recorded continuously throughout this process to produce a load displacement curve form from which the nanomechanical properties such as Young's modulus of elasticity, hardness, fracture toughness, time-dependent creep and plastic and elastic energy of the sample could be calculated [86]. Elastic modulus data may be useful in studies of erosion, since it has been shown to be more sensitive than hardness to the presence of underlying hard material. Indentation depth at some 4,500 µN force in orange juice treated enamel was recorded to be in a range of about 200–500 nm. In comparison, water-treated samples showed indentation depth of 150–350 nm [87]. The nanoindenter could be coupled to the vertical transducer used in combination with AFM, where the cantilever and the laser–optical system is replaced by the transducer–tip system allowing for determination of tip displacements with 0.2 nm resolution [82]. The tip can be scanned across a substrate, building up an image of the area in contact with the tip. Due to the small size of the tip and the indentations with lengths of about 2 µm, the method should be applicable on unpolished samples and for measurements in tiny, defined surface areas.

The nanoindentation method is a very sensitive tool which is able to provide information about material properties.

Element Analysis of Solid Samples

In vitro, trace element analysis of solid tooth samples is feasible with a variety of methods such as, secondary ion mass spectroscopy (SIMS), electron probe microanalysis, laser ablation inductively coupled plasma mass spectroscopy, micro X-ray fluorescence, proton-induced X-ray emission spectroscopy and transmission electron microscopy coupled with a X-ray detection system (Analytical-TEM), laser ablation inductively coupled plasma mass spectroscopy. However, most of these methods are not described for analyzing dental substrates as yet, although they would offer quantitative analysis of elements in very low concentrations in very confined areas of solid samples.

Barbour and Rees [21] described application of SIMS on erosively altered enamel surfaces giving either topographic images or calcium or magnesium surface maps. These images were able to provide information of element loss of the demineralized enamel. The depth of the erosive crater could not be determined with SIMS. Mass spectrometric methods for trace analysis of inorganic materials provide a very sensitive multielemental analysis with limits of detection of low ng g^{-1} concentration range [88]. A broad variety of mass spectrometric methods are described in the literature [89], such as SIMS which allows mono- and multielemental trace analysis on solid materials or thin layers. When solid surfaces are bombarded with ions, these ions penetrate into the solid to a certain depth as a function of their energy and mass and the nature and structure of the sample. The bombarded ions transfer their energy to atoms of the solid. Part of the energy of the primary atoms is returned to the surface of the solid and causes sputtering of neutral particles or secondary ions. With SIMS, the secondary ions mass is analyzed in a mass spectrometer where the ions are separated according to their mass-to-charge ratio giving information about local enrichment or depletion of chemical elements as compared to standard reference materials. However, SIMS is only partially quantitative and actual concentrations cannot be measured accurately.

Electron probe microanalysis is another method establishing the chemical composition of very small volumes of solid material which needs to be polished to a plane surface. The method involves bombarding a specimen with a focused high energy beam of electrons and analyzing the X-ray spectrum emitted from the sample. The X-rays are characteristic of the bombarded elements and allow determination of the quantitative composition of the test samples with wavelength dispersive spectrometers [90]. With sectioned samples element analysis could be performed in subsurface areas with the electron beam hitting the sectioned surface perpendicular to the natural sample surface. Willershausen and Schulz-Dobrick [91] applied this method for evaluating element distribution in sections of eroded enamel in a depth of 5 up to 50 μm. Measurements within the first few micrometers depth of sectioned samples are difficult to perform due to fuzziness at the outermost surface region.

Compared to scanning electron microscopes or transmission electron microscopes equipped with an energy detection system, wavelength dispersive X-ray analyzers in electron probe microanalysis reveals a much higher spectral sensitivity and lower detection limits. Highest lateral resolution (= smallest excited volumes) can be reached with analytical TEM, but this method suffers from the impractical sample preparation of thin specimens and its semiquantitative results.

In summary, element analysis of solid samples allows very sensitive measurements of early mineral loss depending on the method used. However, suitability for erosion assessment has to be checked for most of these methods in the future.

Ultrasonic Measurement of Enamel Thickness

With ultrasonic pulse-echo measurements the time interval between the transmission of an ultrasound pulse on the enamel surface and the echo produced by the amelodentinal junction is determined. Using these data and the mean longitudinal sound velocity in enamel, the thickness of the enamel layer can be calculated. The method is nondestructive allowing in vitro as well as in vivo measurements. It shows good correlation between different operators [92]. However, enamel thickness changes of less than 0.33 mm could not be detected precisely with this method [93] and ultrasonic measurements and histological readings of enamel thickness are only moderately correlated [94].

In table 1, the main advantages and main problems encountered with the described methods are depicted. Moreover, the methods are judged with respect to the requirements, such as their suitability for early erosion or for use with native surfaces. It becomes evident that the complex nature of erosive mineral loss and dissolution might not be comprehended by a single technique, but needs application of different approaches for full understanding. Especially for determination of early erosion, methods with high resolution providing high accuracy might be helpful to gain more insight into the true nature of erosion development as occurring in the oral cavity.

Table 1. Survey of the methods described in detail in the text with respect to main advantages and problems as well as to suitability for use with early erosions (after few minutes of acidic challenge) and with native, nonpolished surface samples

Method	Advantages	Problems	Suitability for early erosion	Suitability for use with native surfaces
SEM and ESEM	– applicable for wet samples (ESEM)	– only qualitative assessment	+	++
Surface hardness measurements	– relatively low costs – long experience – not time-consuming – can be combined with determination of surface loss due to abrasion	– measurement of surface hardness is influenced by nondemineralized deeper layers – polished, flat surfaces needed	++	–
Surface profilometry	– applicable for measurement in natural dentition (replica technique)	– time-consuming when complete mapping of surfaces – stylus could damage surface	–/+	–/+
Iodide permeability test	– low costs	– provides only information about increased pore volumes	–/+	+
Chemical analysis of dissolved minerals	–mostly easy and well-established methods	– no information about structural changes	+++	++
Microradiography	– determination of both mineral loss and demineralization possible	– limited resolution – demanding sample preparation	–	–
Confocal laser scanning microscopy	– high resolution	– only qualitative assessment	++	–/+
Quantitative light-induced fluorescence	– surface scan is not time-consuming	– limited resolution – low experience in erosion studies – exact repositioning of samples for comparative measurements is difficult	–	–

Table 1. (continued)

Method	Advantages	Problems	Suitability for early erosion	Suitability for use with native surfaces
Atomic Force Microscopy	– high resolution – nearly nondestructive	– time-consuming measurement – only limited areas of about 250 × 250 μm could be scanned – high costs	+++	+++
Element analysis of solid samples	– very sensitive (depending on method)	– high costs – highly demanding methods	++(+)	++(+)
Nanoindentation	– very sensitive – provides also information of material properties	– time-consuming measurements – demanding sample preparation	+++	++
Ultrasonic measurement	– allows nondestructive analysis without extensive sample preparation	– low resolution	–	–/+

+++ = Highly suitable; ++ = very suitable; + = suitable; –/+ = limitedly suitable; – = not suitable.

Acknowledgements

The author would like to thank Dr. Wolfgang Buchalla (Department of Operative Dentistry Preventive Dentistry and Periodontology, University of Göttingen) and Dr. Andreas Kronz (Geochemical Institute, University of Göttingen) for critical review of parts of the manuscript.

References

1   Attin T, Buchalla W, Gollner M, Hellwig E: Use of variable remineralization periods to improve the abrasion resistance of previously eroded enamel. Caries Res 2000;34:48–52.
2   Eisenburger M, Hughes J, West NX, Jandt KD, Addy M: Ultrasonication as a method to study enamel demineralisation during acid erosion. Caries Res 2000;34:289–294.
3   Davis WB, Winter PJ: The effect of abrasion on enamel and dentine and exposure to dietary acid. Br Dent J 1980;148:253–256.
4   Attin T, Koidl U, Buchalla W, Schaller HG, Kielbassa AM, Hellwig E: Correlation of microhardness and wear in differently eroded bovine dental enamel. Arch Oral Biol 1997;42:243–250.

5   Smith BGN, Robb ND: Dental erosion in patients with chronic-alcoholism. J Dent 1989;17:219–221.

6   Shah VP, Midha KK, Dighe S, McGilveray IJ, Skelly JP, Yacobi A, Layloff T, Viswanathan CT, Cook CE, McDowall RD: Analytical methods validation: bioavailability, bioequivalence and pharmacokinetic studies. Conference report. Eur J Drug Metab Pharmacokinet 1991;16:249–255.

7   Shah VP, Midha KK, Findlay JW, Hill HM, Hulse JD, McGilveray IJ, McKay G, Miller KJ, Patnaik RN, Powell ML, Tonelli A, Viswanathan CT, Yacobi A: Bioanalytical method validation: a revisit with a decade of progress. Pharm Res 2000;17:1551–1557.

8   Attin T, Becker K, Hannig C, Buchalla W, Hilgers R: A method to detect minimal amounts of calcium in acidic solutions. Caries Res 2005; in press.

9   Koulourides T, Chien MC: The ICT in situ experimental model in dental research. J Dent Res 1992;71 (spec no):822–827.

10 Koulourides T, Phantumvanit P, Munksgaard EC, Housch T: An intraoral model used for studies of fluoride incorporation in enamel. J Oral Pathol 1974;3:185–196.

11 Koulourides T, Volker JF: Changes of enamel microhardness in the human mouth. Ala J Med Sci 1964;35:435–437.

12 Grenby TH: Methods of assessing erosion and erosive potential. Eur J Oral Sci 1996;104: 207–214.

13 West NX, Jandt KD: Methodologies and instrumentation to measure tooth wear; future perspectives; in Addy M, Embery G, Edgar WM, Orchadson R (eds): Tooth Wear and Sensitivity. London, Martin Dunitz, 2000, pp 105–120.

14 Meurman JH, Frank RM: Scanning electron microscopic study of the effect of salivary pellicle on enamel erosion. Caries Res 1991;25:1–6.

15 Hannig M, Balz M: Protective properties of salivary pellicles from two different intraoral sites on enamel erosion. Caries Res 2001;35:142–148.

16 Hannig M, Balz M: Influence of in vivo formed salivary pellicle on enamel erosion. Caries Res 1999;33:372–379.

17 Hannig C, Hamkens A, Becker K, Attin R, Attin T: Erosive effects of different acids on bovine enamel: release of calcium and phosphate in vitro. Arch Oral Biol 2005;50:541–552.

18 Meurman JH, Drysdale T, Frank RM: Experimental erosion of dentin. Scand J Dent Res 1991;99:457–462.

19 Eisenburger M, Shellis RP, Addy M: Scanning electron microscopy of softened enamel. Caries Res 2004;38:67–74.

20 Shellis RP, Hallsworth AS: The use of scanning electron microscopy in studying enamel caries. Scanning Microsc 1987;1:1109–1123.

21 Barbour ME, Rees JS: The laboratory assessment of enamel erosion: a review. J Dent 2004;32: 591–602.

22 Herkströter FM, Witjes M, Ruben J, Arends J: Time dependency of microhardness indentations in human and bovine dentine compared with human enamel. Caries Res 1989;23:342–344.

23 Lussi A, Jaeggi T, Jaeggi-Scharer S: Prediction of the erosive potential of some beverages. Caries Res 1995;29:349–354.

24 Featherstone JD, Ten Cate JM, Shariati M, Arends J: Comparison of artificial caries-like lesions by quantitative microradiography and microhardness profiles. Caries Res 1983;17:385–391.

25 Lussi A, Kohler N, Zero D, Schaffner M, Megert B: A comparison of the erosive potential of different beverages in primary and permanent teeth using an in vitro model. Eur J Oral Sci 2000;108: 110–114.

26 Lussi A, Jaggi T, Scharer S: The influence of different factors on in vitro enamel erosion. Caries Res 1993;27:387–393.

27 Lussi A, Jaeggi T, Zero D: The role of diet in the aetiology of dental erosion. Caries Res 2004;38 (suppl 1):34–44.

28 Jaeggi T, Lussi A: Toothbrush abrasion of erosively altered enamel after intraoral exposure to saliva: an in situ study. Caries Res 1999;33:455–461.

29 Joiner A, Weader E, Cox TF: The measurement of enamel wear of two toothpastes. Oral Health Prev Dent 2004;2:383–388.

30 Joiner A, Pickles MJ, Tanner C, Weader E, Doyle P: An in situ model to study the toothpaste abrasion of enamel. J Clin Periodontol 2004;31:434–438.

31 Lussi A, Jaeggi T, Gerber C, Megert B: Effect of amine/sodium fluoride rinsing on toothbrush abrasion of softened enamel in situ. Caries Res 2004;38:567–571.

32 Schweizer-Hirt CM, Schait A, Schmid R, Imfeld T, Lutz F, Muhlemann HR: Erosion and abrasion of the dental enamel. Experimental study. SSO Schweiz Monatsschr Zahnheilkd 1978;88:497–529.

33 Hooper S, West NX, Sharif N, Smith S, North M, De'Ath J, Parker DM, Roedig-Penman A, Addy M: A comparison of enamel erosion by a new sports drink compared to two proprietary products: a controlled, crossover study in situ. J Dent 2004;32:541–545.

34 Ganss C, Klimek J, Schwarz N: A comparative profilometric in vitro study of the susceptibility of polished and natural human enamel and dentine surfaces to erosive demineralization. Arch Oral Biol 2000;45:897–902.

35 West NX, Hughes JA, Parker DM, Moohan M, Addy M: Development of low erosive carbonated fruit drinks. 2. Evaluation of an experimental carbonated blackcurrant drink compared to a conventional carbonated drink. J Dent 2003;31:361–365.

36 Hughes JA, Jandt KD, Baker N, Parker D, Newcombe RG, Eisenburger M, Addy M: Further modification to soft drinks to minimise erosion. A study in situ. Caries Res 2002;36:70–74.

37 Whitehead SA, Shearer AC, Watts DC, Wilson NHF: Comparison of two stylus methods for measuring surface texture. Dent Mater 1999;15:79–86.

38 Hooper S, West NX, Pickles MJ, Joiner A, Newcombe RG, Addy M: Investigation of erosion and abrasion on enamel and dentine: a model in situ using toothpastes of different abrasivity. J Clin Periodontol 2003;30:802–808.

39 Venables MC, Shaw L, Jeukendrup AE, Roedig-Penman A, Finke M, Newcombe RG, Parry J, Smith AJ: Erosive effect of a new sports drink on dental enamel during exercise. Med Sci Sports Exerc 2005;37:39–44.

40 Attin T, Weiss K, Becker K, Buchalla W, Wiegand A: Impact of modified acidic soft drinks on enamel erosion. Oral Dis 2005;11:7–12.

41 Chadwick RG, Mitchell HL, Cameron I, Hunter B, Tulley M: Development of a novel system for assessing tooth and restoration wear. J Dent 1997;25:41–47.

42 Mitchell HL, Chadwick RG, Ward S, Manton SL: Assessment of a procedure for detecting minute levels of tooth erosion. Med Biol Eng Comput 2003;41:464–469.

43 Mitchell HL, Chadwick RG: Mathematical shape matching as a tool in tooth wear assessment – development and conduct. J Oral Rehabil 1998;25:921–928.

44 Chadwick RG, Mitchell HL, Ward S: Evaluation of the accuracy and reproducibility of a replication technique for the manufacture of electroconductive replicas for use in quantitative clinical dental wear studies. J Oral Rehabil 2002;29:540–545.

45 Chadwick RG, Mitchell HL, Ward S: A novel approach to evaluating the reproducibility of a replication technique for the manufacture of electroconductive replicas for use in quantitative clinical dental wear studies. J Oral Rehabil 2004;31:335–339.

46 Bakhos Y, Brudevold F, Aasenden R: In vivo estimation of the permeability of surface human enamel. Arch Oral Biol 1977;22:599–603.

47 Brudevold F, Tehrani A, Cruz R: The relationship among the permeability to iodide, pore volume, and intraoral mineralization of abraded enamel. J Dent Res 1982;61:645–648.

48 Bakhos Y, Brudevold F: Effect of initial demineralization on the permeability of human tooth enamel to iodide. Arch Oral Biol 1982;27:193–196.

49 Zero DT, Rahbek I, Fu J, Proskin HM, Featherstone JD: Comparison of the iodide permeability test, the surface microhardness test, and mineral dissolution of bovine enamel following acid challenge. Caries Res 1990;24:181–188.

50 Ten Cate JM, Larsen MJ, Pearce EI, Fejerskov O: Chemical interactions between the tooth and oral fluids; in Fejerskov O, Kidd EAM (eds): Dental Caries. The Disease and Its Clinical Management. Copenhagen, Blackwell Munksgaard, 2003, pp 49–70.

51 Hannig M, Hess NJ, Hoth-Hannig W, De Vrese M: Influence of salivary pellicle formation time on enamel demineralization: an in situ pilot study. Clin Oral Investig 2003;7:158–161.

52 van Rijkom H, Ruben J, Vieira A, Huysmans MC, Truin GJ, Mulder J: Erosion-inhibiting effect of sodium fluoride and titanium tetrafluoride treatment in vitro. Eur J Oral Sci 2003;111:253–257.

53 Nekrashevych Y, Stosser L: Protective influence of experimentally formed salivary pellicle on enamel erosion: an in vitro study. Caries Res 2003;37:225–231.

54 Mahoney E, Beattie J, Swain M, Kilpatrick N: Preliminary in vitro assessment of erosive potential using the ultra-micro-indentation system. Caries Res 2003;37:218–224.

55 Grenby TH, Phillips A, Desai T, Mistry M: Laboratory studies of the dental properties of soft drinks. Br J Nutr 1989;62:451–464.

56 Chen PS, Toribara TY, Warner H: Microdetermination of phosphorus. Anal Chem 1956;28: 1756–1758.

57 Lowry OH, Roberts NR, Leiner KJ, Wu ML, Farr L: The quantitative histochemistry of the brain. J Biol Chem 1954;207:1–15.

58 Hohenwallner W, Wimmer E: Malachite green micromethod for determination of inorganic-phosphate. Clin Chim Acta 1973;45:169–175.

59 Hattab F, Linden LA: Micro-determination of phosphate in enamel biopsy samples using the malachite green method. Acta Odontol Scand 1984;42:85–91.

60 Attin T, Becker K, Hannig C, Buchalla W, Wiegand A: Suitability of a malachite green procedure to detect minimal amounts of phosphate dissolved in acidic solutions. Clin Oral Investig 2005;39:432–436.

61 de Josselin de Jong E, van der Linden AH, ten Bosch JJ: Longitudinal microradiography: a nondestructive automated quantitative method to follow mineral changes in mineralised tissue slices. Phys Med Biol 1987;32:1209–1220.

62 de Josselin de Jong E, van der Linden AH, Borsboom PC, ten Bosch JJ: Determination of mineral changes in human dental enamel by longitudinal microradiography and scanning optical monitoring and their correlation with chemical analysis. Caries Res 1988;22:153–159.

63 Anderson P, Elliott JC: Rates of mineral loss in human enamel during in vitro demineralization perpendicular and parallel to the natural surface. Caries Res 2000;34:33–40.

64 Fejerskov O, Nyvad B, Kidd EAM: Clinical and histological manifestations of dental caries; in Fejerskov O, Kidd EAM (eds): Dental Caries. The Disease and Its Clinical Management. Oxford, Blackwell Munksgaard, 2003, pp 71–98.

65 Hall AF, Sadler JP, Strang R, de Josselin de Jong E, Foye RH, Creanor SL: Application of transverse microradiography for measurement of mineral loss by acid erosion. Adv Dent Res 1997;11: 420–425.

66 Amaechi BT, Higham SM, Edgar WM: Use of transverse microradiography to quantify mineral loss by erosion in bovine enamel. Caries Res 1998;32:351–356.

67 Amaechi BT, Higham SM: In vitro remineralisation of eroded enamel lesions by saliva. J Dent 2001;29:371–376.

68 Amaechi BT, Higham SM: Eroded enamel lesion remineralization by saliva as a possible factor in the site-specificity of human dental erosion. Arch Oral Biol 2001;46:697–703.

69 Ganss C, Klimek J, Schaffer U, Spall T: Effectiveness of two fluoridation measures on erosion progression in human enamel and dentine in vitro. Caries Res 2001;35:325–330.

70 Ganss C, Klimek J, Brune V, Schurmann A: Effects of two fluoridation measures on erosion progression in human enamel and dentine in situ. Caries Res 2004;38:561–566.

71 Ganss C, Klimek J, Starck C: Quantitative analysis of the impact of the organic matrix on the fluoride effect on erosion progression in human dentine using longitudinal microradiography. Arch Oral Biol 2004;49:931–935.

72 Ganss C, Lussi A, Klimek J: Comparison of calcium/phosphorus analysis, longitudinal microradiography and profilometry for the quantitative assessment of erosive demineralisation. Caries Res 2005;39:178–184.

73 Duschner H, Sønju-Clasen B, Øgaard B: Detection of early caries by confocal laser scanning microscopy; in Stookey GK (ed): Early Detection of Dental Caries. Indianapolis, Indiana University Press, 1996, pp 145–156.

74 Grotz KA, Duschner H, Reichert TE, de Aguiar EG, Götz H, Wagner W: Histotomography of the odontoblast processes at the dentine-enamel junction of permanent healthy human teeth in the confocal laser scanning microscope. Clin Oral Investig 1998;2:21–25.

75 White DJ, Kozak KM, Zoladz JR, Duschner H, Gotz H: Peroxide interactions with hard tissues: effects on surface hardness and surface/subsurface ultrastructural properties. Compend Contin Educ Dent 2002;23:42–48.

76 Duschner H, Götz H, Walker H, Lussi A: Erosion of dental enamel visualized by confocal laser scanning microscopy; in Addy M, Embery G, Edgar WM, Orchadson R (eds): Tooth Wear and Sensitivity. London, Martin Dunitz, 2000, pp 67–73.

77 Lussi A, Hellwig E: Erosive potential of oral care products. Caries Res 2001;35(suppl 1):52–56.

78 Zentner A, Duschner H: Structural changes of acid etched enamel examined under confocal laser scanning microscope. J Orofac Orthop 1996;57:202–209.

79 van der Veen MH, de Josselin de Jong E: Application of quantitative light-induced fluorescence for assessing early caries lesions; in Faller RV (ed): Assessment of Oral Health: Diagnostic Techniques and Validation Criteria. Basel, Karger, 2000, pp 144–162.

80 Pretty IA, Edgar WM, Higham SM: The erosive potential of commercially available mouthrinses on enamel as measured by quantitative light-induced fluorescence (QLF). J Dent 2003;31:313–319.

81 Pretty IA, Edgar WM, Higham SM: The validation of quantitative light-induced fluorescence to quantify acid erosion of human enamel. Arch Oral Biol 2004;49:285–294.

82 Jandt KD: Atomic force microscopy of biomaterials surfaces and interfaces. Surf Sci 2001;491:303–332.

83 Lippert F, Parker DM, Jandt KD: In vitro demineralization/remineralization cycles at human tooth enamel surfaces investigated by AFM and nanoindentation. J Colloid Interface Sci 2004;280:442–448.

84 Lippert F, Parker DM, Jandt KD: Toothbrush abrasion of surface softened enamel studied with tapping mode AFM and AFM nanoindentation. Caries Res 2004;38:464–472.

85 Finke M, Jandt KD, Parker DM: The early stages of native enamel dissolution studied with atomic force microscopy. J Colloid Interface Sci 2000;232:156–164.

86 Oliver WC, Pharr GM: An improved technique for determining hardness and elastic-modulus using load and displacement sensing indentation experiments. J Mater Res 1992;7:1564–1583.

87 Finke M, Hughes JA, Parker DM, Jandt KD: Mechanical properties of in situ demineralised human enamel measured by AFM nanoindentation. Surf Sci 2001;491:456–467.

88 Lodding AR, Fischer PM, Odelius H, Noren JG, Sennerby L, Johansson CB, Chabala JM, Levisetti R: Secondary ion mass-spectrometry in the study of biomineralizations and biomaterials. Anal Chim Acta 1990;241:299–314.

89 Becker JS, Dietze HJ: Inorganic trace analysis by mass spectrometry. Spectrochim Acta [B] 1998;53:1475–1506.

90 Love G, Scott VD: Electron probe microanalysis using soft X-rays: a review. 1. Instrumentation, spectrum processing and detection sensitivity. J Microsc (Oxf) 2001;201:1–32.

91 Willershausen B, Schulz-Dobrick B: In vitro study on dental erosion provoked by various beverages using electron probe microanalysis. Eur J Med Res 2004;9:432–438.

92 Huysmans MC, Thijssen JM: Ultrasonic measurement of enamel thickness: a tool for monitoring dental erosion? J Dent 2000;28:187–191.

93 Louwerse C, Kjaeldgaard M, Huysmans MC: The reproducibility of ultrasonic enamel thickness measurements: an in vitro study. J Dent 2004;32:83–89.

94 Arslantunali TD, Ozturk F, Lagerweij M, Hayran O, Stookey GK, Caliskan YF: Thickness measurement of worn molar cusps by ultrasound. Caries Res 2005;39:139–143.

Prof. Dr. Thomas Attin
Center for Dental and Oral Medicine and Maxillo-facial Surgery,
University of Zurich
Clinic for Preventive Dentistry, Periodontology and Cariology
Plattenstrasse 11
CH–8032 Zürich

Lussi A (ed): Dental Erosion.
Monogr Oral Sci. Basel, Karger, 2006, vol 20, pp 173–189

Dentine Hypersensitivity

N.X. West

Applied Clinical Research Group, Dental School, Bristol, UK

Abstract

Dentine hypersensitivity is a common oral complaint, affecting the teeth of many individuals. The aetiology is multifactorial; however, over recent years the role of erosion has become more and more important. For dentine hypersensitivity to occur, the lesion must first be localised on the tooth surface and then initiated to exposed dentine tubules which are patent to the pulp. The short, sharp pain symptoms are thought to be derived from the hydrodynamic theory of pain. This episodic pain condition is likely to become a more frequent dental complaint in the future due to the increase in longevity of the dentition and the rise in tooth wear. However, conclusive evidence of successful treatment regimens still eludes us despite a multitude of products available for treatment. In explanation, pain studies are notoriously difficult to conduct due to the subjective nature of pain and the complexity of pain assessment. The basic principles of treatment are altering fluid flow in the dentinal tubules with tubule occlusion or modifying or blocking pulpal nerve response, chemically with agents like potassium or physically.

Dentine hypersensitivity is a common oral complaint, affecting the teeth of many individuals. In the future, it is reasonable to surmise that with the increasing life expectancy of the western population with a functional natural dentition [1] prone to tooth wear, dentine hypersensitivity is likely to become a more frequent dental complaint and an increase in requests for treatment thus follows. Yet, conclusive evidence of successful treatment regimens still eludes us despite a multitude of products available for treatment! The explanation is due to the complexity of pain assessment and the nature of the episodic disease process which will be discussed in this chapter.

Definition and Prevalence

Dentine hypersensitivity is characterised by short, sharp, pain arising from exposed dentine in response to stimuli, typically thermal, evaporative, tactile, osmotic or chemical, which cannot be ascribed to any other form of dental defect or pathology [2]. Great care must be given in diagnosis of the condition to exclude all other dental defects and pathology, as these can give rise to a similar pain [3]. A further small modification to this definition was suggested by the Canadian Advisory Board on Dentine Hypersensitivity in 2003 [4], who suggested that disease should be substituted for pathology.

The pain experienced in dentine hypersensitivity is classically of rapid onset, sharp in character and of the duration of the applied suitable stimulus, although it can persist as a dull throbbing ache for variable periods [5]. The teeth most frequently affected are the buccal, cervical regions of permanent canines and premolars [6], where the enamel tapers at the ameocemental junction. The trigeminal nerve supplies the pulp, with innervation from myelinated fibres, A-β and A-δ, and non-myelinated C fibres [7].

- The larger myelinated fibres (A-β and some A-δ) can respond to stimuli that displace the fluid in the dentinal tubule through a hydrodynamic mechanism such as tactile, evaporative, osmotic or thermal challenges, to elicit short, sharp, stabbing pain that typically lasts for only a few seconds.
- Pulpal C fibres and some of the slowest A-δ fibres appear to respond to intense stimuli that reach the pulp rather than stimulation to dentine surfaces, such as inflammatory conditions like pulpitis or intense heat and chemical stimulation. This pain is a dull, throbbing, aching pain which typically lasts for hours. These nerves are not excited by the hydrodynamic mechanism.

The status of the pulpal fibres in dentine hypersensitivity is not known although symptoms would suggest minor inflammation due to the length of time symptoms persist without developing into a true pulpitis. The terminology of dentine hypersensitivity could therefore be questioned, and indeed the term dentine sensitivity would be more accurate to describe the clinical condition. Another term, root sensitivity, has also been suggested by the 2002 Workshop of the European Federation of Periodontology [8], for dentine hypersensitivity arising from recession in periodontal disease and following periodontal treatment. This group of individuals have micro-organisms invading the root dentinal tubules of periodontally involved teeth [9]. Hence, this condition is of different aetiology but with similar pain symptoms. As the definition of dentine hypersensitivity was developed at an international meeting, it would seem prudent to keep this definition.

Dentine hypersensitivity can present from early teenage to old age, but the majority of sufferers range from 20 to 40 years with a peak in incidence at the end of the third decade [10]. After the age of about 40, aetiological processes tend to mean that the sensitivity reduces due to reparative processes such as secondary dentine which will decrease permeability and reduce the hydraulic conductance of dentine. Females are more frequently affected and at a younger mean age [11, 12], although with any medical condition more females tend to present than males. Different professionals also report different perceived levels of dentine hypersensitivity in their patients, with hygienists reporting twice the level perceived by dentists [4].

Prevalence figures vary from 3 to 57% [10, 11, 13–17]. A figure of 15% is fairly consistently reported when patients were examined by professionals [18].

Differential Diagnosis

There are a number of other dental conditions, which give the same pain symptoms as dentine hypersensitivity. It is therefore essential that a differential diagnosis is made. Other causes of short, sharp dentinal pain include:
- Chipped teeth causing exposed dentine.
- Fractured restorations and incorrectly placed dentine pins.
- Pulpal response to caries and to restorative treatment.
- Inappropriate application of various medicaments during cavity floor preparation.
- Lack of care while contouring restorations so the tooth is left in traumatic occlusion.
- Cracked tooth syndrome, often in heavily restored teeth.
- Palatogingival groove and other enamel invaginations.
- Ditching of margins of amalgam restorations and surface wear on composites.
- Incorrect placement of dentine adhesives in restorative dentistry leading to nanoleakage.
- Caries.
- Vital bleaching.

Pain Mechanism Theories

Various theories have been proposed over the years to explain the pain mechanism of dentinal hypersensitivity:
- Dentinal receptor mechanism.
- Odontoblastic transducer mechanism.
- Nerves in the pulp and not in the dentine are pain receptors:

Nerves stimulated by a hydrodynamic mechanism.

Nerve impulses modulated by the release of polypeptides.

The dentinal receptor mechanism theory implies that dentine hypersensitivity is due to direct stimulation of sensory nerve endings in dentine. Clinicians knew that newly exposed dentine was very sensitive and concluded that the nerve fibres must extend from the pulp into the dentine and may be to the amelodentinal junction. Histologists, however, proved many of theories were false due to the misleading finding that silver staining techniques were not specific, highlighting both reticular and collagen fibres [19]. In conclusion, on the basis of microscopic and experimental data, it seems unlikely that neural cells exist in the sensory portion of the outer dentine. The odontoblast transducer mechanism proposed by Rapp et al. [20] was the sequel theory, suggesting that odontoblasts acted as receptor cells mediating changes in the membrane potential of the odontoblasts via synaptic junctions with nerves. This could result in the sensation of pain from the nerve endings located in the pulpodentinal border. With the evolution of the electron microscope there were misgivings concerning this theory of sensitivity, with failure to demonstrate synaptic complexes between pulpal nerves and odontoblasts, although close contact seemed to exist [21, 22]. In summary, the evidence for the odontoblast transducer mechanism theory is lacking and inconclusive.

The next theory, and one which is supported to date, is the hydrodynamic theory. Brännström [23], working on Gysi's [24] hypothesis that dentine hypersensitivity may be due to movement of the dentinal tubule contents, suggested the hydrodynamic theory of sensitivity. An increased outward fluid flow causes a pressure change across the dentine, distorting the A-δ fibres by a mechanoreceptor action to cause pain. There may be an another process involved, as when fluid flow changes rate in a tubule, there is an electrical discharge called 'streaming potential' across the dentine. This may be able to electrically stimulate nerves.

The width of the tubule is very important, as the rate of fluid flow is dependent on the fourth power of the radius. A doubling of the tubule diameter thus results in a 16-fold increase in fluid flow [25], with sensitive teeth having many more (8×) and wider (2×) tubules at the buccal cervical area compared to non-sensitive teeth. Additionally, dye penetration to the pulp was only seen in sensitive teeth [26]. Further, higher velocity of fluid flow occurs in tubules of smaller diameter, possibly provoking pain sensations.

The poorly localised, dull, burning ache is thought to be due to unmyelinated nerves, C fibres and sympathetic nerves [27]. Vasoactive polypeptides like plasma kinins, calcitonin-gene-related peptide, neurokinins and substance P are found in, e.g., C fibres. After possible injurious stimuli to the odontoblasts, it is possible that polypeptides may be involved in the regulation of neural transmission mediated by the C fibres [28], triggering inflammatory reactions [29], termed 'neurogenic inflammation' [30].

Aetiology

For dentine hypersensitivity to occur, firstly the dentine needs to become exposed (lesion localisation) and secondly the tubules need to be patent to the pulp (lesion initiation). Many young adults have dentine exposed to the oral environment, due to loss of cementum and/or enamel, but clinical experience indicates that only a proportion suffer from dentine hypersensitivity [31]. Any process causing cervical dentine exposure and tubular opening can in theory lead to tooth sensitivity, suggesting a multifactorial aetiology.

Loss of enamel is predominantly a wear process of erosion (intrinsic or extrinsic acids) accompanied by abrasion, attrition or abfraction. Gingival recession is most likely to result from overzealous toothbrushing, periodontal disease, periodontal treatment or trauma, resulting in the dentine being exposed to particularly abrasion and erosion factors. Synergistic action for example between erosion and abrasion forces is highly likely to occur. Following localisation of exposed dentine, it is most likely that initiation is primarily erosion/abrasion based. In vitro studies indicate erosion from acidic soft drinks causes rapid loss of the smear layer to open tubules widely [32], and similarly most toothpastes readily remove the smear layer to expose tubules [32, 33].

Management Strategies for Dentine Hypersensitivity

Clinical experience suggests that the professional approach to treating dentine hypersensitivity has been based on results of treatment rather than addressing the aetiological and predisposing factors, which created the problem. Hence a vast array of products are available to professionals formulated to treat dentine hypersensitivity, many showing equivocal efficacy.

Reviewing dentine hypersensitivity clinical trials helps to explain this conundrum. Protocols for comparing different agents are not standardised, resulting in numerous variables to be compared. A paste with an active agent may be tested against its base paste, a conventional fluoride paste or another paste with an active agent. Treatments rarely take into account aetiological factors, and the measurement of pain is difficult to standardise between individuals due to its subjective nature. Further, complicating factors such as the placebo effect, Hawthorn effect, regression to the mode and control product effect, compound the interpretation of clinical findings and hide the true effect of the treatment. In a study by West et al. [34], the placebo effect was shown to be 40%, reducing the symptom range available to show significance for the agent tested. The clinical efficacy of many of the current products tested also appears to be at the lower end of the therapeutic range. This may be due to low success rate of the agent reaching the target site, lack of sensitivity of the clinical trial, lack of understanding of the patients' interpretation of the pain evoking stimuli, recovery time between repeated stimulation, clinician/patient relationship or indeed the potency of the active agent [35].

Prior to advocating treatment regimens it is important to consider changing aetiological causative agents in order to prevent the perpetuation of the condition. The treatment plan would be as follows:

(1) Confirm the correct diagnosis and exclude the differential diagnoses.

(2) Identify aetiological and predisposing factors particularly in respect of erosion and abrasion with a good dental and medical history and advise accordingly.

(3) Advise on dentine hypersensitivity treatment strategy.

Two treatment modalities are used in the treatment of dentine hypersensitivity, alteration of fluid flow in the tubules and modification or blocking of the pulpal nerve response.

Alteration of Fluid Flow in Dentinal Tubules

Blocking tubules should abolish the sharp, shooting dentinal pain symptoms. The most direct approach to desensitising dentine is occlusion of the tubule orifice. Toothpaste constituents, such as silica abrasives [36] or active agents, have been proposed to occlude tubules. Surface barriers can also be professionally applied in many forms such as varnishes, dentine bonding agents, composite resins, glass ionomer cements and compomers.

The effectiveness of the tubular occluding agents will depend on their resistance to removal. In vitro results demonstrate a number of agents, which can occlude tubules but this does not necessarily correlate to the in vivo situation when there must be resistance to the oral challenges of day-to-day activity. Occluding materials can be washed from the tubule, or may be acid labile. Wear can also occur, abrading the surface of, e.g., a dentine-bonding agent or glass ionomer after a couple of months.

Modification or Blocking of Pulpal Nerve Response
Chemically, e.g. Potassium Ions

Desensitising agents such as potassium ions may reduce intradental nerve excitability by diffusing along the tubules and raising the concentration of local extracellular potassium ions, hence blocking intradental nerve function [37]. This hypothesis is based on animal experiments and has not been confirmed on human teeth where the diffusion distances are greater [38] and where there is a continual outward flow of dentinal fluid to the oral environment [39], which tends to oppose any inward diffusion [40].

Physically, e.g. Endodontics, Extraction
Obviously, these methods are permanently effective at stopping pain from dentine hypersensitivity by removing the nerve or tooth.

Administration of Treatment

Treatment for dentine hypersensitivity can be administered professionally, or for use at home, depending on the degree of the problem and the dentist/patient preference. Home treatment usually involves toothpastes and mouthwashes and is by far the easiest method of administering treatment. It is also fairly inexpensive.

Over-the-Counter Products in the Management of Dentine Hypersensitivity

A wide range of commercially available products are manufactured for self-treatment. Current products in the market place include potassium, strontium, oxalate and fluoride salts combined in toothpastes, gels and mouthrinses.

Strontium Salts
Toothpastes containing strontium salts have dominated the market of desensitising pastes for the last 30 years and have therefore been subjected to most methods of testing for efficacy [41]. In recent years there have been five clinical studies, published between 1992 and 1997 [34, 42–45], investigating the efficacy of strontium compounds in toothpastes for the treatment of dentine hypersensitivity, 3 applying strontium chloride and 3 strontium acetate. Comparison between these studies is hindered by the variation in protocol procedures and toothpaste formulation investigated. Overall, the studies demonstrated an improvement in patients' perception of pain; however, it is important to compare inter- not intragroup differences. Further, the effectiveness of the product at reducing symptoms appears to increase with increased usage [46]. In conclusion, analyses of these studies demonstrate strontium salts have equivocal beneficial effects at reducing dentine hypersensitivity under these trial designs.

The theory behind incorporating strontium salts in toothpastes derives from the ability of the salt to have a considerable affinity for dentine owing to the high permeability and possibility for absorption into or onto the organic connective tissues and the odontoblast processes [47]. It has been proposed that strontium combines with dentine to form a strontium apatite complex with a significantly higher radiodensity than hydroxyapatite [48]. Kun [49] conducted a radiolabelled study attempting to demonstrate topical strontium chloride hexahydrate toothpaste produced a deposit of strontium on the dentine surface, but tubular occlusion could not be substantiated by this methodology. Another theory postulated for the therapeutic action of the strontium-based pastes is the possible effect of the abrasive fillers. Work in vitro with the strontium acetate toothpaste has been very promising, achieving good tubule occlusion of etched dentine due to the silica abrasive [33, 36, 50]. Even more exciting was the finding that the silica layer was not removed on rinsing [50]. Unfortunately, these properties have not been demonstrated clinically with the same success as in the treatment of dentine hypersensitivity.

Potassium Salts

Potassium salts are now the most commonly used agents for the treatment of dentine hypersensitivity being incorporated into toothpastes and mouthrinses. The most frequently used potassium salts are nitrates, chloride, citrates and oxalates. A number of studies have investigated potassium salts [34, 44, 45, 51–56], with results showing an improvement in the patients' perceived symptoms of dentine hypersensitivity. Further and more importantly, studies on toothpastes by a number of authors have demonstrated a significant benefit from a potassium-based paste over a control paste [45, 51, 53, 54], although other studies failed to show these beneficial effects [34, 44]. Much of the early work testing potassium nitrate employed an electrical stimulus as a quantitative variable [57–59]. This stimulus, however, has been questioned as an unnatural stimulus representing the pain of dentine hypersensitivity.

The implication of the placebo effect must not be underestimated with the control product showing efficacy. This is clearly demonstrated in the [60] study.

In addition to the possible mechanisms already mentioned for the action of potassium ions, citrates have the ability to chelate calcium. Hence, it is possible that tubular occlusion may occur, resulting in the reduction of pain due to dentine hypersensitivity.

Very few studies have evaluated active agents in mouthrinses and 2 of these have both potassium salts [44, 60]. Neither of these well-designed studies demonstrated efficacy of the potassium nitrate or citrate agent, respectively.

Particular attention has been focused on potassium nitrate including a Cochrane review [61]. Due to the rigour of this type of systematic review, which included a meta-analysis, very few (only four) of the published papers in this field could be incorporated. Consequentially, the reviewers concluded that there was no strong evidence available to support the efficacy of potassium nitrate for the treatment of dentine hypersensitivity. This reiterates the need to look carefully at trial design for future studies to achieve more meaningful data.

Oxalates

The idea of oxalates acting as desensitising agents has gained popularity. The mode of action has been proposed as tubule occlusion by oxalate ions reacting with calcium ions in the dentinal fluid to form insoluble calcium oxalate crystals, 1–2 μm in diameter, deposited in the tubule apertures [62]. This was confirmed by Mongiorgi and Prati [63], with X-ray diffractometer analysis. A recent in vitro study by Suge et al. [64] evaluated the effects of pre- or post-application of calcium chloride on enhancing the occluding ability of potassium oxalate. However, results showed no significant treatment effect due to calcium-enhanced uptake. In vitro work has shown that while oxalates result in good tubule occlusion, they are acid labile and can be easily washed from the surface of dentine [36].

The oxalate salts commonly used in commercially available products are potassium, citrate, ferric, dipotassium and monohydrogen–monopotassium [65] found that dipotassium oxalate produced fewer but significantly larger calcium oxalate crystals than monohydrogen–monopotassium oxalate; however, the larger crystals were not as effective at occluding the open tubules. Monohydrogen–monopotassium oxalate also had a pH lower than dipotassium oxalate, 3 vs. 5.6, respectively, and therefore the former released a much higher concentration of calcium ions from dentine and accelerated crystal formation. In summary, oxalates appear to have limited ability to reduce the pain from dentine hypersensitivity.

Fluorides

Incorporation of fluoride in the majority of toothpastes is now favoured by most oral health care companies, due to its proven beneficial effects on reduction of caries. Various fluoride compounds have been documented for the treatment of dentine hypersensitivity; these include sodium fluoride, sodium silico-fluoride, stannous fluoride and sodium monofluorophosphate.

It has been suggested that fluoride may eventually mechanically block the tubules, or labile fluoride in the organic matrix of the dentine blocks the transmission of stimuli. The former view would support Brännström's [23] hydrodynamic theory and was also favoured by Greenhill and Pashley [62]. Stannous fluoride, although demonstrating some efficacy in reducing dentine hypersensitivity, has a major disadvantage in that it stains teeth and margins of restorations. More recent findings suggest that sodium fluoride is superior to sodium monofluorophosphate regarding fluoride deposition on the teeth [66]. It is interesting to note that dentine hypersensitivity is still a large problem where populations use fluoridated toothpaste and live in fluoridated water regions. This may be due to the delivery system [2]. The majority of toothpastes now contain fluoride in some form, as do many mouthwashes. There are also specifically designed mouthwashes and toothpastes for high fluoride uptake, yet still the incidence of dentine hypersensitivity is high.

Sodium Citrate Pluronic F-127 Gel

Sodium citrate pluronic F-127 gel has been shown to significantly reduce the hydraulic conductance of dentine in vitro [62]. According to the Council on Dental Therapeutics, USA [67], a toothpaste containing 2% dibasic sodium citrate pluronic F-127 gel is a safe and effective form of treatment in controlling dentine hypersensitivity. However, as with potassium nitrate, there are equivocal data.

Other Agents

The effectiveness of a home use dental rinse containing aluminium lactate was compared to the control rinse of Higuchi et al. [68] with some success.

Professionally Applied Products in the Management of Dentine Hypersensitivity

Again, a wide range of commercially available products is available for professional treatment. In-office treatments tend to be reserved for the individuals who have received preventive advice and have tried products for home use but found them ineffective.

Varnishes and Precipitants

Professionally applied sodium fluoride has been used to treat dentine hypersensitivity [69]. A varnish can set by releasing ethanol and taking up moisture. In this way, the insoluble resins in the shape of a sticky-plastic congealing film gradually fall out, e.g., sodium fluoride is thought to dissolve and deposit on the tooth. Observation shows that this approach reduces the pain of dentine hypersensitivity for as long as it stays on the tooth. Although several authors demonstrate a distinct enrichment of the surface enamel with such a varnish [70, 71], it may be that the varnish is effective due to occlusion of the tubules by the resin rather than to the effect of the fluoride. A calcium/fluoride solution is currently marketed which also contains silica, giving good clinical results.

Oxalates like fluoride have also been applied professionally; however, success rates for efficacy are equivocal.

Other Treatment Modalities

Alternative treatment regimens include those of Chinese traditional medicine, which are becoming more and more popular in the Western world, particularly when treatment fails by orthodox methods. Dentine hypersensitivity has been treated successfully in China by brushing teeth with a mixture of root Dahurian, angelica, the root of Chinese wild ginger, puncture vine, the rhizome of davallia, peppermint and gallnut [72]. Unfortunately, no clinical trials have yet been undertaken.

Calcium hydroxide was a popular agent for the treatment of dentine hypersensitivity [73–75]. Trowbridge [5] failed to come to this conclusion when testing cat canine teeth, calcium hydroxide being insoluble and not able to release many free calcium ions. This agent is rarely used today.

Studies involving the use of corticosteriods have provided little evidence of efficacy, and their use is based on the assumption that hypersensitivity is linked to pulpal inflammation which has not been proved. Other out-dated forms of treatment for dentine hypersensitivity includes application of silver nitrate, zinc chloride and formalin.

Restorative Materials

Glass ionomer, resin-reinforced glass ionomer/compomers, adhesive resin primers and adhesive resin bonding systems have been used successfully for the treatment of dentine hypersensitivity. Treatment can be problematic if there has been little tissue loss and over contouring can lead to plaque retentive sites and gingival inflammation [76]. Further, suffers of dentine hypersensitivity tend to be meticulous at cleaning their teeth, often using excessive brushing force on frequent occasions. Unless the toothbrushing habits are corrected, materials can be abraded and need replacement.

Low [77] evaluated glass ionomers in the treatment of this condition with a good success rate; however, evaluation of pain was not described. Hansen [78] has also reported success using resin-reinforced glass ionomer. Cavity varnish can give temporary relief of symptoms when applied in a thin film on open dentinal tubules [79]; however, the smear layer must be modified or removed before application in order to occlude the tubules and be stable to acidic attack.

The use of adhesive resin primer products are documented in vitro to occlude tubules [80], and clinically by Ianzano et al. [81]; however, there were no untreated control teeth in the trial. Other groups [82] could not demonstrate efficacy clinically. In theory, the concept is clear and practical, with the thin films occluding the tubules. However, sometimes failure of polymerisation occurs and the films can be easily abraded.

Dondi dall'Orologio et al. [83] concluded following testing a primer and conditioner that both were highly effective in reducing or eliminating dentine sensitivity for periods up to 6 months. A study by Martens [84] agreed with these findings; however, if the seal between the material and the root surface brakes down, dentine sensitivity may reoccur. The systems incorporating the primer and adhesive components together produce a thicker film and have been used with success [85]. A well-controlled study by Ide et al. [86] using another commercially available system again gave good efficacy, the surface not being etched prior to application of material. The latest hydrophilic bonding systems are designed to provide a better bond in a wet environment.

In conclusion, these materials are frequently used by clinicians for the treatment of dentine hypersensitivity. There are few well-controlled trials to support their efficacy. Those which have been reported together with clinical experience would support the use of these materials after employment of preventive advice and home use treatment, particularly for isolated teeth that have not responded.

Lasers

Nd:YAG laser irradiation has been advocated for the alleviation of symptoms from dentine hypersensitivity. They are thought to work by coagulation of proteins in the dentinal fluid and hence reduce permeability [87]. They are also believed to create an amorphous sealed layer on the dentine surface which appears to be due to partial melt down of the surface [88]. However, there is a possibility that the peripheral tubules are opened, negating any benefit. The Nd:YAG laser has been used with encouraging results [89, 90]. Other clinical studies do not support this finding [91], with the laser treatment reducing the pain sensation but not significantly different from the placebo treatment.

Recently, the GaAlAs laser was compared to a fluoride varnish in a clinical trial [92] with no significant differences found, and an Er:YAG laser [93] showed some effect compared to the control at low setting.

In summary, the clinical results obtained from laser therapy are equivocal and do not seem to justify the high expenditure of the equipment for this purpose.

Iontophoresis

Iontophoresis is another method that has been investigated for the treatment of dentine hypersensitivity. The mechanism is thought to enhance fluoride uptake possibly by activating tertiary dentine formation [94]. However, a more likely explanation is an increased reduction to acid decalcification and or precipitations in the open tubules, due to the presence of fluoride [95, 96]. Iontophoresis is technically difficult and very operator sensitive, as the current can easily pass through the gingivae instead of the dentine [97]. Jensen [13] reported excellent results using an iontophoretic toothbrush with a toothpaste containing 2,000 ppm of sodium fluoride. Gangarosa et al. [98] and Lutins et al. [99] conducted double-blind trials and Carlo et al. [100] open ones, using iontophoresis with topical application of 2% sodium fluoride, with immediate success. Ideally, well-controlled clinical trials are needed; however, there is no substantial explanation for the effect, if any, of iontophoresis.

Periodontal Surgery

Coronally repositioning periodontal flaps to cover areas of exposed dentine has been advocated as a treatment regimen for dentine hypersensitivity [101]. Compared to the other modalities of treatment for this condition this is an invasive procedure and results can be unpredictable due to further recession occurring in the area.

Endododontics and Extraction of Teeth

As a last resort these treatment procedures have been used to alleviate the pain of dentine hypersensitivity when all other methods of pain relief fail.

Conclusion

Clinically, there are many treatment modalities for dentine hypersensitivity which the clinician finds successful to alleviate the pain of dentine hypersensitivity. If one toothpaste is not found to be effective another may be used with success. Hence, the patient needs to try a number of different approaches. Unfortunately, no one treatment seems to suit all. The least invasive treatments are usually advocated first followed by the professional led treatment.

In recent years, the standard of reporting in clinical trials has improved, particularly with the advent of good clinical practice [102], and yet unequivocal data on efficacy of products for the treatment of dentine hypersensitivity have not been produced, despite sound theory, in vitro data and supporting clinical trials. Attention must therefore be focused on the design of the clinical trial in order to perfect a model that can differentiate between products and accommodate challenges such as the placebo effect.

References

1   Nuttall N, Steele JG, Nunn J, Pine C, Treasure E, Bradnock G, Morris J, Kelly M, Pitts NB, White D: A guide to the UK Adult Dental Health Survey 1998. London, British Dental Association, 2001, pp 1–6.
2   Dowell P, Addy M: Dentine hypersensitivity: a review, aetiology, symptoms and theories of pain production. J Clin Periodontol 1983;10:341–350.

3   Dowell P, Addy M, Dummer P: Dentine hypersensitivity: aetiology, differential diagnosis and management. Br Dent J 1985;158:92–96.

4   Canadian Advisory Board on Dentine Hypersensitivity: Consensus-based recommendations for the diagnosis and management of dentine hypersensitivity. J Can Dent Assoc 2003;69:221–228.

5   Trowbridge HO: Mechanism of pain induction in hypersensitive teeth; in Rowe NH (ed): Proceedings of Symposium on Hypersensitive Dentine: Origin and Management. 1985, p 1.

6   Orchardson R, Collins WJN. Clinical features of hypersensitive teeth. Br Dent J 1987;162: 253–256.

7   Matthews B, Andrew D, Wanachantararak S. Biology of the dental pulp with special reference to its vasculaure and innervation; in Addy M, Embery G, Edgar WM, Orchardson R (eds): Tooth Wear and Sensitivity. London, Martin Dunitz, 2000, pp 39–51.

8   Sanz M, Addy M: Group D summary. J Clin Periodontol 2002;29(suppl 3):195–196.

9   Adriaens PA, DeBoever JA, Loesche WJ. Bacterial invasion in root, cementum and radicular dentine of periodontally diseased teeth in humans: a reservoir of periodontopathic bacteria. J Periodontol 1988;59:222–230.

10   Graf HE, Galasse R: Morbidity, prevalence and intra-oral distribution of hypersensitive teeth. J Dent Res 1977;56:abstr 479.

11   Flynn N, Galloway R, Orchardson R: The incidence of hypersensitive teeth in the West of Scotland. J Dent 1985;13:230–236.

12   Addy M, Mostafa P, Newcombe RG: Dentine hypersensitivity: a comparison of five toothpastes used during a 6-week period. Br Dent J 1987;163:45–50.

13   Jensen AL: Hypersensitivity controlled by iontophoresis: double blind clinical investigation. J Am Dent Assoc 1964;68:216–225.

14   Iwrin CR, McCusker P: Prevalence of dentine hypersensitivity in general population. J Ir Dent Assoc 1997;43:7–9

15   Murray LE, Roberts AJ: The prevalence of reported hypersensitive teeth. Arch Oral Biol 1994;39(suppl):129S.

16   Rees JS: The prevalence of dentine hypersensitivity in general practice in the UK. J Clin Periodontol 2000;27:860–865.

17   Lui H, Lan WH, Hsieh CC: Prevalence and distribution of cervical dentine hypersensitivity in a population in Taipai, Taiwan. J Endod 1998;24:45–47.

18   Fischer C, Fischer RG, Wennberg A: Prevalence and distribution of cervical dentine hypersensitivity in a population in Rio de Janeiro, Brazil. J Dent 1992;20:272–276.

19   Rapp R, Avery JK, Rector RA: A study of the distribution of nerves in human teeth. J Can Dent Assoc 1957;23:447–453.

20   Rapp R, Avery JK, Strachen DS: Possible role of the aceylcholinesterase in neural conduction within the dental pulp; in Finn SB (ed): Biology of Dental Pulp Organ. Birmingham, University of Alabama Press, 1968, p 309.

21   Byers MR: Dental sensory receptors. Int Rev Neurobiol 1984;25:39.

22   Holland GR: The odontoblast process: form and function. J Dent Res 1985;64:499–514.

23   Brännström M: A hydrodynamic mechanism in the transmission of pain-produced stimuli through the dentine; in Anderson DJ (ed): Sensory Mechanisms in Dentine. New York, Pergamon Press 1963, pp 73–79.

24   Gysi A: An attempt to explain the sensitiveness of dentin. Br J Dent Sci 1900;43:865–868.

25   Guyton A: Textbook of Medical Physiology, ed 4. Philadelphia, Saunders, 1971, pp 211–212.

26   Absi EG, Addy M, Adams D: Dentine hypersensitivity: a study of the patency of dentinal tubules in sensitive and non sensitive cervical dentine. J Clin Periodontol 1987;14:280–284.

27   Närhi MVO: Dentine sensitivity: a review. J Biol Buccale 1985;13:75–96.

28   Närhi MVO, Hiroven T, Hakumähi M: Responses of intradental nerve fibres to stimulation of dentine and pulp. Acta Physiol Scand 1982;115:173–178.

29   Pashley DH: Mechanisms of dentine sensitivity. Dent Clin N Am 1990;34:449–474.

30   Lisney SJW, Bharali AM: The axon reflex: an outdated idea of a valid hypothesis? News Physiol Sci 1989;4:45.

31   Addy M, Mostafa P, Newcombe RG: Dentine hypersensitivity: the distribution of recession, sensitivity and plaque. J Dent 1987;15:242–248.

32   Absi EG, Addy M, Adams D: Dentine hypersensitivity the effects of toothbrushing and dietary compounds on dentine in vitro: a SEM study. J Oral Rehabil 1992;19:101–110.

33   West NX: Dentine hypersensitivity: clinical and laboratory studies of toothpastes, their ingredients and acids, PhD, University of Wales,1995.

34   West NX, Addy M, Jackson RJ, Ridge DB: Dentin hypersensitivity and the placebo respons: a comparison of the effect of strontium acetate, potassium nitrate and fluoride toothpastes. J Clin Periodontol 1997;24:209–215.

35   Curro FA, Friedman M, Leight RS: Design and conduct of clinical trials on dentine hypersensitivity; in Addy M, Embery G, Edgar WM, Orchardson R (eds): Tooth Wear and Sensitivity. London, Martin Dunitz, 2000, pp 300–314.

36   Addy M, Mostafa P: Dentine hypersensitivity. 11. Effects produced by the uptake in vitro of toothpastes onto dentine. J Oral Rehab 1989;16:35–48.

37   Markowitz K, Bilotto G, Kim S: Decreasing intradental nerve activity in the cat with potassium and divalent cations. Arch Oral Biol 1991;36:1–7.

38   Peacock JM, Orchardson R: Effects of potassium ions on action potential conduction in A- and C-fibers of rat spinal nerves. J Dent Res 1995;74:634–641.

39   Vanuspong W, Eisenburger M, Addy M: Cervical tooth wear and sensitivity: erosion, softening and rehardening of dentine: effects of pH, time and ultrasonication. J Clin Periodontol 2002;29: 351–357.

40   Pashley DH, Matthews WG: The effects of outward forced connective flow on inward diffusion in human dentine in vitro. Arch Oral Biol 1993;38:557–582.

41   Kanapka JA: Over the counter dentifrices in the treatment of tooth hypersensitivity: review of clinical studies. Dent Clin N Am 1990;34:545–560.

42   Gillam DG, Newman HN, Davies EH, Bulman JS: Clinical efficacy of a low abrasive dentifrice for the relief of cervical dentinal hypersensitivity. J Clin Periodontol 1992;19:197–201.

43   Pearce NX, Addy M, Newcombe RG: Dentin hypersensitivity: a clinical trial to compare 2 strontium desensitising toothpastes with conventional fluoride toothpaste. J Periodontol 1994;65: 113–119.

44   Gillam DG, Bulman JS, Jackson RJ, Newman HN: Efficacy of a potassium nitrate mouthwash in alleviating cervical dentine hypersensitivity. J Clin Periodontol 1966;23:993–997.

45   Silverman G, Bermal E, Hanna CB: Assessing the efficacy of three dentifrices in the treatment of dentinal hypersensitivity. J Am Dent Assoc 1996;127:191–201.

46   Jackson RJ: Potential treatment modalities for dentine hypersensitivity; in Addy M, Embery G, Edgar WM, Orchardson R (eds): Tooth Wear and Sensitivity. London, Martin Dunitz, 2000, pp 327–338.

47   Ross MR: Hypersensitive teeth: effect of strontium chloride in a compatible dentifrice. J Periodontol 1961;32:49–53.

48   Gedalia I, Brayer L, Kalter N: The effect of fluoride and strontium application on dentine: in vivo and in vitro studies. J Periodontol 1978;49:269–272.

49   Kun L: Etude biophysique des modifications des tissues dentaires prevoquees par l'application totale de Strontium. Schweiz Monatschr Zahnheilk 1976;86:661–676.

50   Banfield N, Addy M: Dentine hypersensitivity: development and evaluation of a model in situ to study tubule patency. J Clin Periodontol 2004;31:325–335.

51   Salvato AR, Clark GE, Gingold J, Curro FA: Clinical effectiveness of a dentifrice containing potassium chloride as a desensitising agent. Am J Dent 1994;5:303–306.

52   Nagata T, Ishida H, Shinohara H, Nishikawa S, Kasahara S, Wakano Y, Daigen S, Troullos ES: Clinical evaluation of a potassium nitrate dentifrice for the treatment of dentine hypersensitivity. J Clin Periodontol 1994;21:217–221.

53   Silverman G, Gingold J, Curro FA: Desensitising effect of a potassium chloride dentifrice. Am J Dent 1994;7:9–12.

54   Schiff T, Dotson M, Cohen S: Efficacy of a dentifrice containing potassium nitrate, soluble pyrophosphate, PVM/MA copolymer, and sodium fluoride on dentinal hypersensitivity: a twelve-week clinical study. J Clin Dent 1994;5:87–92.

55   Ayad F, Berta R, De Vizio W, Volpe A: Comparative efficacy off two dentifrices containing 5% potassium nitrate on dentinal sensitivity: a twelve-week clinical study. J Clin Dent 1994;5:97–101.

56 Chesters R, Kaufman HW, Wolff MS, Huntington E, Kleinber GI: Use of multiple sensitivity measurements and logit statistical analysis to assess the effectiveness of a potassium-citrate-containing dentifrice in reducing dentinal hypersensitivity. J Clin Periodontol 1992;19:256–261.

57 Tarbet WJ, Silverman G, Stolman JM, Fratarcangelo PA: An evaluation of two methods for the quantitation of dentinal hypersensitivity. J Am Dent Assoc 1979;98:914–918.

58 Tarbet WJ, Silverman G, Stolman JM, Fratarcangelo PA: Clinical evaluation of a new treatment for dentinal hypersensitivity. J Periodontol 1980;51:535–540.

59 Tarbet W, Silverman G, Fratarcangelo PA , Kanapka JA: Home treatment for dentinal hypersensitivity: a comparative study. J Am Dent Assoc 1982;105:227–230.

60 Yates R, West NX, Addy M, Marlow I: The effects of a potassium citrate, cetylpyridium chloride, sodium fluoride mouthrinse on dentin hypersensitivity, plaque and gingivitis. J Clin Periodontol 1998;25:813–820.

61 Poulsen S, Errboe M, Hovgaard O, Worthington HW: Potassium Nitrate Toothpaste for Dentine Hypersensitivity (Cochrane Review) From The Cochrane Library. Chichester, Wiley, 2005.

62 Greenhill JD, Pashley DH: Effects of desensitizing agents on the hydraulic conductance of human dentine in vitro. J Dent 1981;60:686–698.

63 Mongiorgi R, Prati C: Mineralogical and crystallographical study of γ-calcium oxalate on dentine surfaces in vitro. Arch Oral Biol 1994;39(suppl):152.

64 Suge I, Kawasski A, Ishikawa K, Matsuo I, Ebisu S: Effects pre-or post application of calcium chloride on occluding ability of potassium oxalate for the treatment of dentine hypersensitivity. Am J Dent 2005;18:121–125.

65 Pashley DH, Galloway SE: The effects of oxalate treatment on the smear layer of ground surfaces of human dentine. Arch Oral Biol 1985;30:731–737.

66 Duckworth RM, Moore SS: Salivary fluoride clearance after use of NaF dentifrices: a dose response study. J Dent Res 1994;73:abstr 263.

67 Council on Dental Therapeutic: Accepted Dental Therapeutics, ed 40. Chicago, American Dental Association, 1984, p 421.

68 Higuchi Y, Kurihara H, Nishimura F, Miyamoto M, Arai H, Nakagawa M, Murayama Y, Suido H, Tanii S: Clinical evaluation of a dental rinse containing aluminium lactate for the treatment of dentine hypersensitivity. J Clin Dent 1996;7:9–12.

69 Clark DC, Hanley JA, Geoghegan S: The effectiveness of a fluoride varnish and a desensitizing toothpaste in treating dentine hypersensitivity. J Dent Res 1985;20:212.

70 Petersson LG: Fluoride gradients outermost surface enamel after varied forms of topical application of fluorides in vivo. Odontologisk Revy 1976;27:25.

71 Arends J, Lodding A, Petersson LG: Fluoride uptake in enamel. Caries Res 1980;14:403.

72 Zhang H-Q, Wu XB: Treatment of dentin hypersensitivity with Chinese traditional medicines. Hypersensitive Dentine: Biological Basis of Therapy IADR/AADR Satellite Symposium 1993, p 33. Arch Oral Biol 1994;39:136S.

73 Levin MP, Yearwood LL, Carpenter WN: The desensitizing effect of calcium hydroxide and magnesium hydroxide on hypersensitive dentine. Oral Surg Oral Med Oral Pathol 1973;35:741–746.

74 Jorkjend L, Tronstad L: Treatment of hypersensitive root surfaces by calcium hydroxide. Scand J Dent Res 1972;80:264–266.

75 Green BL, Green ML, McFall WT: Calcium hydroxide and potassium nitrate as desensitizing agents for hypersensitive root surfaces. J Periodontol 1977;48:667–672.

76 Trowbridge HO, Silver DR: A review of current approaches to in-office management of tooth hypersensitivity. Dent Clin N Am 1990;34:561–582.

77 Low T: The treatment of hypersensitive cervical abrasion cavities using ASPA cement. J Oral Rehabil 1981;8:81–89.

78 Hansen EK: Dentine hypersensitivity treated with a fluoride containing varnish or a light cures glass ionomer liner. Scand J Dent Res 1992;100:305–309.

79 Hack GH, Thompson VP: Cavity varnishes: their ability to occlude dentinal tubules. Hypersensitive dentine: biological basis of therapy. IADR/AADR Satellite Symposium 1993, p 46. Arch Oral Biol 1994;39:149S.

80 Simpson ME, Ciarlone AE, Pashley DH: Effects of dentine primers on dentine permeability. J Dent Res 1993;72:127, abstr 185.

81   Ianzano JA, Gwinnet AJ, Westbay G: Polymeric sealing of dentinal tubules to control sensitivity: preliminary observations. Periodontal Clin Investig 1993;15:13–16.

82   Anderson MH, Powell LV: Desensitization of exposed dentin using a dentine bonding system. J Dent Res 1994;73:297, abstr 1559.

83   Dondi dall'Orologio GD, Borghetti R, Calicetic C, Lorenzi R, Malferrari S: Clinical evaluation of Gluma and Gluma 2000 for treatment of hypersensitive dentine. Arch Oral Biol 1994;39 (suppl):126.

84   Martens LC: Effects of anti-sensitive toothpaste on opened dentinal tubules and on two dentin-bonded resins. Clin Prev Dent 1991;13:23–28.

85   Russell CM, Dickinson GL, Downey MC: One-step versus Protect in the treatment of dentinal hypersensitivity. J Dent Res 1997;77:199, abstr 748.

86   Ide M, Morel AD, Wilson RH, Ashley FP: The role of a dentine bonding agent in reducing cervical dentine sensitivity. J Clin Periodontol 1998;25:286–290.

87   Goodis HE, White JM, Marshall SJ, Marshall GW: Laser treatment of sensitive dentine. Arch Oral Biol 1994;39(suppl):128.

88   Matsumoto K, Funai H, Wakabayashi H, Oyoama T: Study of the treatment of hypersensitive dentine by GaAIAs laser diode. Jpn J Conserv Dent 1985;28:54.

89   Renton-Harper P, Midda M: ND YAG laser treatment of dentinal hypersensitivity. Br Dent J 1992;172:13–26.

90   Lan WH, Lui HC: Treatment of dentine hypersensitivity by Nd:YAG laser. J Clin Laser Med Surg 1996;14:89–92.

91   Lier BB, Rosing CK, Aass AM, Gjermo P: Treatment of dentine hypersensitivity by Nd:YAG laser. J Clin Periodontol 2002;29:501–506.

92   Corona SA, Nascimento TN, Catirse AB, Lizarelli RF, Dinelli W, Palma-Dibb RG: Clinical evaluation of low-level therapy and fluoride varnish for treating cervical dentinal hypersensitivity J Oral Rehabil 2003;30:1183–1189.

93   Schwartz F, Arweiler N, Georg T, Reich E: Desensitising effects of an Er:YAG laser on hypersensitive dentine. J Clin Periodontol 2002;29:211–215.

94   Schaeffer ML, Bixler D, Pao-Lo Y: The effectiveness of iontophoresis in reducing cervical hypersensitivity. J Periodontol 1971;42:695.

95   Selvig KA: Ultrasonic changes in human dentine exposed to weak acid. Arch Oral Biol 1968;13:719–734.

96   Furseth R: A study of experimentally exposed and fluoride treated dental cementum in pigs. Acta Odontol Scand 1970;28:833–850.

97   Ciancio SG: Delivery systems and clinical significance of available agents for dentinal hypersensitivity. Endodont Dent Traumatol 1986;2:150–152.

98   Gangarosa LP, Buettner AL, Baker WP, Buettner BK, Thompson WO: Double-blind evaluation of duration of dentin sensitivity reduction by iontophoresis. J Gen Dent 1989;37:316–319.

99   Lutins ND, Greco GW, McFall WT: Effectiveness of sodium fluoride on tooth hypersensitivity with and without ionophoresis. J Periodontol 1984;55:285.

100 Carlo GT, Ciancio SG, Seyrek SK: An evaluation of iontophoretic application of fluoride for tooth desensitisation. J Am Dent Assoc 1982;105:452–454.

101 Lindhe J: Clinical Periodontology and Implant Dentistry, ed 3. Copenhagen, Munksgaard,1998, p 569.

102 ICH Topic 6 Guideline for Good Clinical Practice: CPMP/ICH/135/95 17th July, 1996.

Dr. N.X. West
Restorative Dentistry (Perio)
University of Bristol Dental Hospital and School
Lower Maudlin Street
Bristol BS1 2LY (UK)

Lussi A (ed): Dental Erosion.
Monogr Oral Sci. Basel, Karger, 2006, vol 20, pp 190–199

··········•············

Risk Assessment and Preventive Measures

A. Lussi[a], *E. Hellwig*[b]

[a]Department of Preventive, Restorative and Pediatric Dentistry, School of Dental Medicine, University of Bern, Bern, Switzerland; [b]Department of Operative Dentistry and Periodontology, University Clinic of Dentistry, Freiburg, Germany

Abstract

A prerequisite for preventive measures is to diagnose erosive tooth wear and to evaluate the different etiological factors in order to identify persons at risk. No diagnostic device is available for the assessment of erosive defects. Thus, they can only be detected clinically. Consequently, erosion not diagnosed in the early stage may render timely preventive measures difficult. In order to assess the risk factors, patient should record their dietary intake for a distinct period of time. Then a dentist can determine the erosive potential of the diet. Particularly, patients with more than four dietary acid intakes have a higher risk for erosion when other risk factors (such as holding the drink in the mouth) are present. Regurgitation of gastric acids (reflux, vomiting, alcohol abuse, etc.) is a further important risk factor for the development of erosion which has to be taken into account. Based on these analyses, an individually tailored preventive program may be suggested to the patients. It may comprise dietary advice, optimization of fluoride regimes, stimulation of salivary flow rate, use of buffering medicaments and particular motivation for nondestructive toothbrushing habits with a low abrasive toothpaste. The frequent use of fluoride gel and fluoride solution in addition to fluoride toothpaste offers the opportunity to reduce somewhat abrasion of tooth substance. It is also advisable to avoid abrasive tooth cleaning and whitening products, since they may remove the pellicle and may render teeth more susceptible to erosion. Since erosion, attrition and abrasion often occur simultaneously all causative components must be taken into consideration when planning preventive strategies.

The early clinical differentiation of the various defects found under the umbrella of tooth wear (abrasion, attrition, erosion) is important to adequately prevent each of these dental hard tissue defects [1]. The prevention of predominantly abrasion lesions such as wedge-shaped defects, has to be different from prevention of erosive tooth wear. A prerequisite in prevention of above all is the identification of those patients who are at risk of dental erosion in order to initiate primary preventive measures. It is important to evaluate the different etiological factors that may lead to erosion in order to identify persons at risk from erosion. Several predictors have been suggested such as: vomiting and regurgitation, misuse of acidic dietary products, use of acidic medicaments, occupation, use of illegal drugs, lactovegetarian diet, and excessive toothbrushing [2]. These causes and risk factors have been discussed extensively in other chapters and are only covered here when they are of special interest concerning the preventive approach.

Clinical detection of dental erosion is important once dissolution has started. However, there is no diagnostic device available for early clinical detection and quantification of dental erosion. Therefore, the clinical appearance is the most important sign for dental professionals to diagnose erosion. This is of particular importance in the early stages of erosive tooth wear. The appearance of smooth silky-glazed enamel, intact enamel along the gingival margin and grooving on occlusal surfaces are some typical signs of early enamel erosion. It is a difficult task to diagnose erosion at an early stage and it seems to be difficult to assess whether dentine is exposed or not [3]. Therefore, a modern preventive strategy needs training of dentists in early detection and monitoring of the process (see chapter 4 by Ganss et al., this vol, pp 32–43). Only with these capabilities can dentists comply with their responsibilities for providing adequate care for patients. Often patients themselves do not seek treatment until the condition is at an advanced stage or when the teeth become hypersensitive or when the aesthetics are affected. This is particularly true for patients who suffer from anorexia nervosa or bulimia.

When dental erosion is detected by a dentist or when there are indications for an increased risk, detailed patient assessment should be undertaken. All of the causes discussed in the earlier chapters have to be taken into account. A very important part of the patient assessment is case history taking. However, chair-side interviews are generally not sufficient to determine dietary habits that may lead to erosion because the patients may be unaware of their acid ingestion. It is therefore advisable to have such patients record their complete dietary intake for 4 consecutive days (table 1). The time of day and quantity of all ingested foods and beverages including dietary supplements should be recorded. Both weekdays and weekends should be included, as dietary habits during weekends may be considerably different from those during weekdays. This dietary and behavior record should be sent to the dentist prior to the next appointment. The dentist should determine the erosive potential of the different acidic food items and drinks, the frequency of ingestion during main meals and snacks, and is then able to estimate the daily acid challenge. Erosion protecting

Table 1. Example of a patient's dietary history (to be recorded over 4 consecutive days including a weekend)

Time	Foods/beverages, method of drinking	Oral hygiene
Day 1, Date: 06.06.2006		
6.30	Yoghurt, 1 apple, honey, coffee with milk	Toothbrushing immediately
9.30	300 ml orange juice, sipping	afterwards
13.00	Cooked whole potatoes, cheese, salad with French dressing, herbal tea and 1 apple	Toothbrushing immediately afterwards
16.15	300 ml orange juice, sipping	Toothbrushing immediately
19.00	Mixed salad with French dressing, bread and herbal tea	afterwards
20.00–21.00	300 ml orange juice, sipping	
22.00	1 acidic candy	
23.00		Toothbrushing

food should also be considered. The erosive potential of certain drinks or foods can be estimated using the information provided earlier (see chapter 7.1.1 by Lussi et al., this vol, pp 77–87).

The progression of erosion seems to be greater in older (52–56 years) compared to younger (32–36 years) persons and has a skewed distribution. One-third of the persons account for more than two-thirds of the total progression [1]. The group with high erosion progression was found to have four or more dietary acid intakes per day, a low buffering capacity of their stimulated saliva and used a hard bristle toothbrush. Intake frequency of the same magnitude was also associated with an increased risk of erosion in children. In this study, the group with erosion ate fruit significantly more frequently and had different drinking habits, such as swishing, sucking or holding drinks in their mouths [4]. The drinking method (holding, sipping, gulping, nipping, sucking) strongly affected tooth-surface pH. It follows that holding or long-sipping of erosive beverages should be avoided, as it causes low pH values for a long period of time [5]. Knowing that in the presence of other risk factors, four or more nutritional acidic intakes per day are associated with higher risk for the development and progression of erosion, assists the dentist in the assessment of the patient [1, 4]. Every patient should be questioned and examined using the information provided in table 2. It has to be kept in mind that acidic lozenges and herbal teas may have an erosive potential and aggravate erosive lesions [6–9]. Possible intrinsic acid exposure should also be taken into account. Based on these analyses, an appropriate preventive program may be suggested to patients (table 3). However, the advice has to be made on an individual basis, so not all points

Table 2. Parameters to be covered in order to unveil etiological factors for erosions (in part from [17])

- Case history (medical and dental)
- Detection of the main noncarious hard tissue lesions (site-specific distribution)
- Record of dietary intake over 4 days (estimation of the erosive potential)
  Specific factors which the patients may not be aware of

Diet	herbal teas, acidic candies, alcohol, sports drinks, effervescent vitamin C tablets, etc
Gastric symptoms	vomiting, acid taste in the mouth and gastric pain (especially when awakening), stomach ache, any sign of anorexia nervosa
Drugs	alcohol, tranquillizer, anti-emetics, anti-histamines, lemonade tablets (change of acidic or saliva-reducing drugs is possible)
- Determination of flow rate and buffering capacity of saliva
- Oral hygiene habits (technique, abrasivity of toothpaste)
- Occupational exposure to acidic environments
- X-ray therapy of the head area
- Silicone impressions, study models, and/or photographs to assess further progression

Table 3. Recommendations for patients at high risk for dental erosion (modified from [17, 37])

- Reduce acid exposure by reducing the frequency, and contact time of acids (main meals only)
- Avoid acidic foods and drinks last thing at night
- Do not hold or swish acidic drinks in your mouth; avoid sipping these drinks; use a straw, ensuring the flow is not aimed directly at any individual tooth surface
- Avoid toothbrushing immediately *after* an erosive challenge (vomiting, acidic diet). Instead, use a fluoride containing mouth rinse, a sodium bicarbonate (baking soda) solution, milk or food such as cheese or sugar-free yoghurt; if none of the above are possible, rinse with water
- Avoid toothbrushing immediately *before* an erosive challenge, as the acquired pellicle provides protection against erosion
- Use a soft toothbrush and low abrasion fluoride containing toothpaste; high abrasive toothpastes may destroy the pellicle; avoid toothpastes or mouthwashes with a too low pH
- Gently apply periodically concentrated topical fluoride (slightly acidic formulations are preferable as they form CaF_2 with a higher rate)
- Consider using modified acid beverages with no or reduced erosive potential
- After acid intake, stimulate saliva flow with chewing gum or lozenges; the use of a non-acidic sugar-free lozenge may be more advisable, since gum chewing may have an abrasive effect on softened tooth structure
- Use chewing gum to reduce postprandial reflux
- Refer patients or advise them to seek appropriate medical attention when intrinsic causes are involved (gastroenterologist and/or a psychologist) (patients with intrinsic erosion)

listed in table 3 are of interest to every patient. The aim of this program is to reduce acid exposure by decreasing the frequency of ingestion of potentially harmful drinks and foodstuffs as well as minimizing contact time with the teeth, and by rapid consumption of them rather than sipping or swishing. In addition, reflux/vomiting should be controlled and the patient's fluoride regime should be optimized. As discussed previously, various processes cause the degradation of tooth substance. Erosion, attrition and abrasion often occur simultaneously, though usually one of these factors may be predominant. When giving preventive instructions, all of the causative components must be taken into consideration. Other behavior that either stimulates salivary flow such as chewing gum or nonacidic lozenges, or that directly helps to neutralize acids such as rinsing with sodium bicarbonate may counter the destructive effects of dietary acids [10, 11]. Patients suffering from intrinsic erosions, depending on the cause, need further care such as antacids, psychological therapy or even surgical intervention. Adequate preventive measures will often slow down progression of the erosion and reduce the need for immediate restorations. However, assessment of erosion change is important – photographs and study casts are simple means of monitoring progression.

Acid-eroded enamel is more susceptible to abrasion and attrition than intact enamel. The thickness of the softened enamel that is removed following different abrasive procedures varies in different investigations depending on the experimental conditions [12–17].

In the 1970s, Graubart et al. [18] showed a protective effect of a 2% sodium fluoride solution in the in vitro erosive process. Less wear of softened teeth was produced in vitro in the presence of fluoride toothpaste than in the presence of nonfluoride toothpaste with an otherwise identical formulation [19]. In recent years, more studies using different fluoride formulations, e.g. sodium fluoride, acidulated phosphate fluoride, stannous fluoride, amine fluoride or titanium tetrafluoride showed a protective effect in vitro [20–23]. Stannous fluoride showed better protection than sodium fluoride when teeth were immersed in 0.1 M HCl with a pH of 2.2. However, when the pH was further lowered to 1.2 (which is lower than the acid content of the stomach) there was no protection [23]. Titanium fluoride was found to be a more effective pretreatment agent against citric acid erosion when compared with sodium fluoride [21]. It appears that in vitro, highly concentrated fluoride gels demonstrated the best protection against further erosion/abrasion. In our own experiments [24], the impact of different fluoride procedures on the prevention of toothbrush abrasion in situ was compared prior to and after the enamel was softened. The softening treatment comprised of application of 0.1 M citric acid (pH 3.5) for 3 min in vitro. Each protocol included four tooth slabs attached to intraoral appliances. After exposing the tooth slabs to the oral milieu for 60 min, the samples

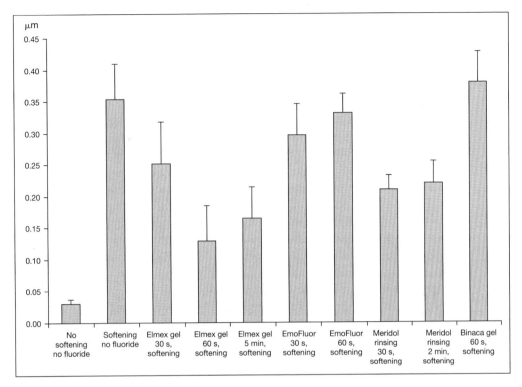

Fig. 1. Mean loss of polished enamel after 15 s toothbrushing in situ (in part from [24]). (1) No softening, no fluoride (control 1); (2) softening, no fluoride (control 2); (3) application of a slightly acidic sodium/amine fluoride gel (Elmex gel, 12,500 ppm F⁻) for 30 s before softening; (4) application of sodium/amine fluoride gel (Elmex gel, 12,500 ppm F⁻) for 1 min before softening; (5) application of sodium/amine fluoride gel (Elmex gel, 12,500 ppm F⁻) for 5 min before softening; (6) application of stannous fluoride (EmoFluor, 1,000 ppm F⁻) for 30 s before softening; (7) application of stannous fluoride (EmoFluor, 1,000 ppm F⁻) for 1 min before softening; (8) rinsing in situ with a stannous/amine fluoride rinsing solution (Meridol rinsing solution, 250 ppm) for 30 s before softening; (9) rinsing in situ with a stannous/amine fluoride rinsing solution (Meridol rinsing solution, 250 ppm) for 2 min before softening; (10) application of a neutral NaF gel (Binaca, 12,500 ppm F⁻) for 1 min before softening.

were brushed for 15 s with medium abrasive toothpaste in situ (fig. 1). The loss of tooth substance was determined, as described earlier [14]. The least amount of toothbrush abrasion occurred when using the slightly acidic sodium/amine fluoride gel for 1 min before softening the enamel, when compared to all of the other experimental groups. There was, however, only partial protection. This was shown earlier when a slightly acidic gel (pH 4.5) showed a greater reduction of abrasion compared to a neutral fluoride gel [25]. This could be as a result of some incorporation of material into and/or deposition of material on the enamel surface, most probably as a CaF_2-like material [20], which will lead to less softening than without this layer. This CaF_2-like layer is considered stable at a neutral pH, but may dissolve as the pH drops during erosive attacks. This deposited CaF_2-like layer may be dissolved readily by most acidic beverages [26, 27].

Until now, only case reports or in situ studies have been undertaken. Jensen et al. [28] published a case report investigating the importance of fluoride in maintaining the dentition. In this study, teeth were obtained from a deceased anorexic and bulimic patient. Just prior to death, saliva analyses and enamel biopsies were made, before and after a 3-week regimen of daily rinsing with 0.05% NaF. Further to 4 years of daily regurgitation there was an almost normal thickness of the enamel present on the palatal surfaces of the anterior teeth, with normal hardness measurements 10 μm away from the outer surface. SEM micrographs showed an irregular topography, with crystalline deposits rich in calcium, phosphate and fluoride. The tooth surfaces exposed to gastric juice were more reactive to uptake of additional fluoride when given as a daily rinse, than the more protected surfaces. This case report suggests that frequent daily use of fluoride products can minimize the erosive effect of gastric contents on tooth enamel. Ganss et al. [29] showed in an in situ model that treatments with fluoridated toothpaste + F solution + slightly acidic F gel could significantly reduce tooth erosion by 50 and 90% on enamel and 10 and 55% on dentine, respectively. Lussi et al. [30] studied in situ, the effect of fluoride rinsing on the prevention of toothbrush abrasion of softened enamel. A single rinse with sodium/amine fluoride solutions before or after erosion had no significant effect on subsequent abrasion by toothbrushing for 30 s. From the above it is clear that further in situ studies are needed. The compliance for restrictive regimes as mentioned above [29] needs very motivated and dedicated patients. It has to be determined whether such strict regimes are feasible in daily practice.

Exposure to saliva has been shown to be effective for rehardening eroded enamel. The mechanism for this is thought to be that once the erosive agent is neutralized or cleared from the tooth surface, the deposition of salivary calcium and phosphate may lead to rehardening of the acid-softened enamel [10, 31]. Enamel specimens eroded by citric acid for 2 h were immersed in artificial saliva and showed partial rehardening after 1–4 h. These specimens remineralized for 6–24 h and demonstrated complete rehardening [32]. Saliva is an important biological factor in the prevention of erosion. It has been speculated that saliva stimulation will enhance the formation of the acquired salivary pellicle. It is known that the pellicle forms rapidly and has some protective effect against erosion [33–36]. Any procedure that removes or reduces the thickness of the salivary pellicle may compromise its protective properties and therefore accelerate the erosion process. Procedures such as toothbrushing with abrasive dentifrice products, professional cleaning with prophylaxis paste, and tooth whitening will all remove or weaken the pellicle and may render teeth more susceptible to erosion [37]. Acidic beverages may interfere with the pellicle formation and thus further modify the protective barrier [38].

As previously discussed, various processes may cause degradation of the tooth substance. When giving preventive instructions, all of the causative components must be taken into consideration. Other behaviors that either stimulate salivary flow (such as chewing gum), or directly help neutralize acids (such as rinsing with sodium bicarbonate), may counter the destructive effects of dietary acids [10, 11]. There is the possibility that chewing gum may have an abrasive effect on softened tooth structure. However, chewing gum after a meal helps to reduce postprandial esophageal acid exposure [39]. It was also suggested that chewing gum might be a treatment option for some patients with symptomatic reflux [40, 41].

For individuals who are at high risk for erosive tooth wear and those with active erosion, it is suggested that toothbrushing should be postponed after consumption of erosive foodstuffs or beverages, in order to minimize enamel loss. Another possibility is to gently apply fluoride prior to the erosive attack. This has to be achieved carefully so that the protecting pellicle is not disturbed. For subjects prone to caries, the risk of enhancing the progression of carious lesions by postponing toothbrushing may be too great following the rapid decrease in plaque pH after ingestion of sugar-containing foods or beverages. Measures that are beneficial for both erosion and caries are rinsing with fluoride solutions, thereby enhancing remineralization and stimulating salivary secretion. The gentle use of nonacidic, saliva-stimulating lozenges may be preferable to chewing gum because it may have an abrasive effect on softened dental hard tissue [37]. Adhesive systems may protect dentine from acid actions and brushing abrasion for a limited period of time [42–44]. There is clearly a need for improvement and development of substances with a high protective capacity against the erosive/abrasive insult.

References

1   Lussi A, Schaffner M: Progression of and risk factors for dental erosion and wedge-shaped defects over a 6-year period. Caries Res 2000;34;182–187.
2   Amaechi BT, Higham SM: Dental erosion: possible approaches to prevention and control. J Dent 2005;33:243–252.
3   Ganss C, Klimek J, Lussi A: Accuracy and consistency of the visual diagnosis of exposed dentine on worn occlusal/incisal surfaces. Caries Res; in press.
4   O'Sullivan EA, Curzon MEJ: A comparison of acidic dietary factors in children with and without dental erosion. J Dent Child 2000;67:186–192.

5   Johansson AK, Lingström P, Imfeld T, Birkhed D: Influence of drinking method on tooth-surface pH in relation to dental erosion. Eur J Oral Sci 2004;112:484–489.

6   Lussi A, Portmann P, Burhop B: Erosion on abraded dental hard tissues by acid lozenges: an in situ study. Clin Oral Investig 1997;1:191–194.

7   Behrendt A, Oberste V, Wetzel EK: Fluoride concentration and pH of iced tea products. Caries Res 2002;36:405–410.

8   Phelan J, Rees J: The erosive potential of some herbal teas. J Dent 2003;31:241–246.

9   Jensdottir T, Nauntofte B, Buchwald C, Bardow A: Effects of sucking acidic candy on whole-mouth saliva composition. Caries Res 2005;39:468–474.

10 Amaechi BT, Higham SM: Eroded lesions remineralisation by saliva as a possible factor in the site – specificity of human dental erosion. Arch Oral Biol 2001;46:697–703.

11 Amaechi BT, Higham SM, Edgar WM: Influence of abrasion in clinical manifestation of human dental erosion. J Oral Rehabil 2003;30:407–413.

12 Davis WB, Winter PJ: The effect of abrasion on enamel and dentine after exposure to dietary acid. Br Dent J 1980;148:253–256.

13 Kelly MP, Smith BGN: The effect of remineralizing solutions on tooth wear in vitro. J Dent Res 1988;16:147–149.

14 Jaeggi T, Lussi A: Toothbrush abrasion of erosively altered enamel after intraoral exposure to saliva: an in situ study. Caries Res 1999;33:455–461.

15 Attin T, Buchalla W, Gollner M, Hellwig E: Use of variable remineralization periods to improve the abrasion resistance of previously eroded enamel. Caries Res 2000;34:48–52.

16 Attin T, Knofel S, Buchalla W, Tutuncu R: In situ evaluation of different remineralization periods to decrease brushing abrasion of demineralized enamel. Caries Res 2001;35:216–222.

17 Lussi A, Jaeggi T, Zero D: The role of diet in the aetiology of dental erosion. Caries Res 2004;38:34–44.

18 Graubart J, Gedalia I, Pisanti S: Effects of fluoride pretreatment in vitro on human teeth exposed to citrus juice. J Dent Res 1972;51:1677.

19 Bartlett DW, Smith BG, Wilson RF: Comparison of the effect of fluoride and non-fluoride toothpaste on tooth wear in vitro and the influence of enamel fluoride concentration and hardness of enamel. Br Dent J 1994;176:346–348.

20 Ganss C, Klimek J, Schäfer U, Spall T: Effectiveness of two fluoridation measures on erosion progression in human enamel and dentine in vitro. Caries Res 2001;35:325–330.

21 van Rijkom H, Ruben J, Vieira A, Huysmans M-CDNJM, Truin G-J, Mulder: Erosion-inhibiting effect of sodium fluoride and titanium tetrafluoride in vitro. Eur J Oral Sci 2003;111:253–257.

22 Hughes JA, West NX, Addy M: The protective effect of fluoride treatments against enamel erosion in vitro. J Oral Rehabil 2004;31:357–363.

23 Willumsen T, Øgaard B, Hansen BF, Rølla G: Effects from pretreatment of stannous fluoride versus sodium fluoride on enamel exposed to 0.1 or 0.01 M hydrochloric acid. Acta Odontol Scand 2004;62:278–281.

24 Lussi A, Jaeggi T, Schaffner M: Prevention and minimally invasive treatment of erosions. Oral Health Prev Dent 2004;2:321–325.

25 Attin T, Deifuss H, Hellwig E: Influence of acidified fluoride gel on abrasion resistance of eroded enamel. Caries Res 1999;33:135–139.

26 Larsen MJ: Prevention by means of fluoride of enamel erosion as caused by soft drinks and orange juice. Caries Res 2001;35:229–234.

27 Larsen MJ, Richards A: Fluoride is unable to reduce dental erosion from soft drinks. Caries Res 2002;36:75–80.

28 Jensen OE, Featherstone JD, Stege P: Chemical and physical oral findings in a case of anorexia nervosa and bulimia. J Oral Pathol 1987;16:399–402.

29 Ganss C, Klimek J, Brune V, Schurmann A: Effects of two fluoridation measures on erosion progression in human enamel and dentine in situ. Caries Res 2004;38:561–566.

30 Lussi A, Jaeggi T, Gerber C, Megert B: Effect of amine/sodium fluoride rinsing on toothbrush abrasion of softened enamel in situ. Caries Res 2004;38:567–571.

31 Gedalia I, Dakuar A, Shapira L, Lewinstein I, Goultschin J, Rahamim E: Enamel softening with Coca-Cola and rehardening with milk or saliva. Am J Dent 1991;4:120–122.

32   Eisenburger M, Addy M, Hughes JA, Shellis RP: Effect of time on the remineralisation of enamel by synthetic saliva after citric acid erosion. Caries Res 2001;35:211–215.

33   Nieuw Amerongen AV, Oderkerk CH, Driessen AA: Role of mucins from human whole saliva in the protection of tooth enamel against demineralization in vitro. Caries Res 1987;21:297–309.

34   Meurman JH, Frank RM: Scanning electron microscopic study of the effect of salivary pellicle on enamel erosion. Caries Res 1991;25:1–6.

35   Hannig M, Balz M: Influence of in vivo formed salivary pellicle on enamel erosion. Caries Res 1999;33:372–379.

36   Hannig M, Fiefiger M, Guntzer M, Dobert A, Zimehl F, Nekrashevych Y: Protective effect of the in situ formed short-term salivary pellicle. Arch Oral Biol 2004;49:903–910.

37   Zero T, Lussi A: Erosion – chemical and biological factors of importance to the dental practitioner. Int Dent J 2005;55:285–290.

38   Finke M, Parker DM, Jandt KD: Influence of soft drinks on the thickness and morphology of in situ acquired pellicle layer on enamel. J Colloid Interface Sci 2002;251:263–270.

39   Avidan B, Sonnenberg A, Schnell TG, Sontag SJ: Walking and chewing reduce postprandial acid reflux. Aliment Pharmacol Ther 2001;15:151–155.

40   von Schonfeld J, Hector M, Evans DF, Wingate DL: Oesophageal acid and salivary secretion: is chewing gum a treatment option for gastro-oesophageal reflux? Digestion 1997;58:111–114.

41   Smoak BR, Koufman JA: Effects of gum chewing on pharyngeal and esophageal pH. Ann Otol Rhinol Laryngol 2001;110:1117–1119.

42   Azzopardi A, Bartlett DW, Watson TF, Sherriff M: The measurement and prevention of erosion. J Dent 2001;29:395–400.

43   Azzopardi A, Bartlett DW, Watson TF, Sherriff M: The surface effects of erosion and abrasion on dentine with and without a protective layer. Br Dent J 2004;196:351–354.

44   Schneider F, Hellwig E, Attin T: Einfluss von Säurewirkung und Bürstabrasion auf den Dentinschutz durch Adhäsivsysteme. Dtsch Zahnärztl Z 2002;57:302–306.

Prof. Dr. Adrian Lussi
Department of Preventive, Restorative and Pediatric Dentistry
School of Dental Medicine
University of Bern, Freiburgstrasse 7
CH–3010 Bern (Switzerland)

Lussi A (ed): Dental Erosion.
Monogr Oral Sci. Basel, Karger, 2006, vol 20, pp 200–214

....

Restorative Therapy of Erosion

Thomas Jaeggi, Anne Grüninger, Adrian Lussi

Department of Preventive, Restorative and Pediatric Dentistry,
School of Dental Medicine, University of Bern, Bern, Switzerland

Abstract

When substance loss caused by erosive tooth wear reaches a certain degree, oral rehabilitation becomes necessary. Prior to the most recent decade, the severely eroded dentition
could only be rehabilitated by the provision of extensive crown and bridge work or removable
overdentures. As a result of the improvements in composite restorative materials, and in
adhesive techniques, it has become possible to rehabilitate eroded dentitions in a less invasive manner. However, even today advanced erosive destruction requires the placement of
more extensive restorations such as ceramic veneers or overlays and crowns. It has to be kept
in mind that the etiology of the erosive lesions needs to be determined in order to halt the disease, otherwise the erosive process will continue to destroy tooth substance. This overview
presents aspects concerning the restorative materials as well as the treatment options available to rehabilitate patients with erosion, from minimally invasive direct composite reconstructions to adhesively retained all-ceramic restorations. Restorative treatment is dependent
on individual circumstances and the perceived needs and concerns of the patient. Long-term
success is only possible when the cause is eliminated. In all situations, the restorative preparations have to follow the principles of minimally invasive treatment.

Early Diagnosis and Prevention

In order to plan adequate preventive and therapeutic measures, a thorough
case history and diagnosis of each patient is mandatory.

The teeth of all patients who are scheduled for a recall appointment, children as well as adults, should not only be examined for caries and periodontal
diseases but also for noncarious tooth surface loss. Special consideration
should be given to the following: dietary habits, drinking habits, sports activities, bad taste in the mouth (especially in the morning), gastric or esophageal
problems. Furthermore, the salivary flow rates and its buffering capacity should

be measured. Patients with presumption of reflux or vomiting problems require to be referred to a gastroenterologist for further examination. If erosive tooth wear is diagnosed at an early stage it may be possible to protect the permanent dentition against further damage. Local preventive measures can enhance remineralization and the acid resistance of enamel and dentine surfaces and provide some protection against erosive challenge [1, 2]. Systemic preventive measures and/or interventions by a gastroenterologist should keep the situation under control and prevent the process from progressing. For more information see chapter 12 by Lussi et al., (this vol, pp 190–199).

Morphological Conditions and Restorative Materials

Initially, erosive tooth wear is limited to the enamel. At this stage of the erosive process, the teeth are not hypersensitive. Restorations may be inserted because of esthetic needs and/or to prevent further progression. Direct composite coatings or in more advanced cases, porcelain veneers should be considered as the treatment of choice. This seals the enamel and reestablishes the tooth contour and minimizes further enamel loss by acid exposure.

In advanced cases, dentine becomes exposed. If dentinal tubules are opened, dentine hypersensitivity can occur (see chapter 11 by West, this vol, pp 173–189). There are different reasons for treatment need: (1) The structural integrity of the tooth is threatened. (2) The exposed dentine is hypersensitive. (3) The erosive defect is esthetically unacceptable to the patient. (4) Pulpal exposure is likely to occur [3]. A clinically correct diagnosis of the condition is essential to manage the adhesion of the restorative material. It was shown that resin bond strengths to noncarious sclerotic cervical dentine are lower than bonding to normal dentine. This is thought to be a result of tubule occlusion by mineral salts, preventing resin tag formation [4]. Ogata et al. [5] investigated the influence of the direction of tubules on bond strength to dentine. They found that for different adhesive systems, a higher tensile bond strength was obtained when tubules were parallel to the bonded interface than when tubules were cut perpendicularly. In another study, the effect of different burrs on dentine bond strengths of self-etching primer bonding systems was evaluated. It was shown that pretreatment of regular dentine with a fine-cut, fissure steel burr showed the best results, followed by a cross-cut fissure steel burr and a diamond burr [6]. Van Dijken [7] investigated the durability of three simplified adhesive systems in cervical abrasion/erosion lesions with dentine involvement. Results showed cumulative loss rates for the 3 systems after 2 years as follows: Clearfil Liner Bond 2 (Kuraray, Okayama, Japan) 9%, One Coat Bond (Coltène, Altstätten, Switzerland) 13%, and Prompt-L-Pop (3M Espe, Seefeld, Germany)

21%. The loss rates of the materials in sclerotic versus nonsclerotic lesions were not significantly different. Restorations placed on diamond burr-roughened lesions showed no difference in retention time when compared to the nonroughened lesions after a 2-year clinical examination period.

Longevity of Restorative Materials and Acidic Conditions

The longevity of dental restorations depends on the durability of the material per se and its wear resistance [8], the durability of the interface between tooth substance and restoration, the level of tooth destruction, its location and load.

In a study, three glass-ionomer restorative materials used for cervical erosion/abrasion lesions were evaluated clinically after 10 years. The authors concluded that when a noninvasive approach is desired, glass-ionomer materials are the restorative material of choice for this kind of lesion because of their long-term retention values [9]. It has to be kept in mind that at the time of this study total-etch dentinal adhesive systems were still improving and hardly any system showed, clinically, restoration margins free of microleakage for an extended time [10]. Gaengler et al. [11] evaluated the longevity of posterior glass-ionomer cement/composite restorations after an examination period of 10 years. They found that the early risk of failure was attributed to bulk fractures and partial loss of filling material. The maximum longevity was a maximum of 74% over 10 years. It was concluded that this form of posterior restoration was clinically appropriate because a high percentage of restorations had correct anatomical form and demonstrated a low secondary caries rate. Future treatment regimes have been made possible by the development of sophisticated preparation techniques, improved adhesive systems and restorative materials that will result in the therapy of more small-sized lesions rather than large restorations. Indirect inlay techniques will shift towards direct restorative techniques. As the cavities become smaller, it is to be expected that the use of improved direct restorative materials will provide excellent longevity even in load-bearing situations [12].

However, it has to be considered that these conclusions were derived from evidence for posterior restorations further to dental caries rather than erosive tooth wear. The chemical degradation of tooth substance and restorative materials as a result of acids may continue, even if preventive measures are initiated. There are different methods that can be used to evaluate the erosion of dental materials: (1) a solubility test; (2) a method that measures the residual weight of a solution in which the dental material has been immersed; (3) a test which measures the depth loss of the material in a cavity filled with it [13]. In such a study [13], the erosion rate of three different types of cement (zinc phosphate, polycarboxylate and glass-ionomer) were evaluated by measuring the depth loss of the cement. Results showed increasing depth losses with increasing immersion period either in a lactic acid solution (pH 2.74) or in a lactic acid/sodium lactate buffer solution (pH 2.74). The depth losses of all cements were considerably more in the buffer solution than in the acid solution and were most for polycarboxylate followed by zinc phosphate and glass ionomer cement. Knobloch et al. [14] investigated the acid solubility and sorption of different resin-based luting cements. Acid solubility was performed in 0.01 M lactic acid. The weight changes of the cements after immersion in distilled water or lactic acid were measured. Significant differences were found among several cements tested for each of the properties investigated. Due to their hydrophilic nature, all resin-modified glass-ionomer cements showed significantly higher water sorption values compared to composite cements. The effect of a carbonated beverage on the wear of human enamel opposed by dental ceramics was measured. Tooth against ceramic specimens were tested in a wear machine in a cycling model with intermittent immersion in Coca-Cola. It was concluded that exposure to the beverage accelerated the enamel wear and decreased the wear resistance of the ceramics [15]. Another study investigated the chemical degradation of composite restorations after conditioning in artificial saliva and various food-simulating liquids for 1 week by measuring the change in surface hardness and the thickness of the degradation layer. Specimens were immersed either in distilled water, 0.02 N citric acid, 0.02 N lactic acid, heptane or in 75–25% ethanol–water solution. The effects of chemical media on hardness change were found to be material dependent. A significant but weak correlation was detected between change in hardness and thickness of the degradation layer [16]. Shabanian and Richards [17] measured, in vitro, the wear rates of dental materials under different loads and varying pH. The three test materials were more resistant than enamel to acid, with the composite demonstrating the lowest susceptibility to acid. The acid and load resistance of the tested resin-modified glass-ionomer cement was less than that of the composite and greater than that of the conventional glass-ionomer cement. Studying the effect of different storage media upon the surface micromorphology of resin-based restoratives, it was found that the surface roughness of restoratives was significantly higher after a pH cycling regime than after storage either in distilled water or in artificial saliva [18]. There are some indications that the dentine–adhesive interface after an acid–base challenge can lead to a degradation [19]. The effect of dietary acids on surface microhardness of various restoratives was measured by Gomec et al. [20]. Specimens were stored in bidistilled water for 1 week and then immersed for another week in aqueous solutions of lactic, orthophosphoric, citric or acetic acid. Results showed that the surface microhardness of the tested materials varied not only with the pH but also with the nature of the acidic solution and the composition of the evaluated material. Citric and acetic acids reduced microhardness, whereas lactic and orthophosphoric acids increased the microhardness of Fuji IX GP (GC America, Alsip, Ill., USA) and Vitremer (3M Espe, Seefeld, Germany); all acidic media reduced the microhardness of Dyract AP (Dentsply DeTrey, Konstanz, Germany) and Prodigy (Kerr, West Collins, Orange, Calif., USA). The interaction of dental restorative materials with acidic beverages has been studied by immersion, with the aim of investigating how long-term contact affects solution pH and specimen surface hardness. All materials were found to reduce the pH of the 0.9% NaCl solution (control) but to increase the pH of the acidic beverages. The conventional glass ionomer dissolved completely in apple and orange juice but survived in Coca-Cola despite, after 1 year immersion time, a significant hardness reduction occurred. The resin-modified glass-ionomers and the compomers survived in apple and orange juice, but showed greater reductions in surface hardness in these beverages than in Coca-Cola. Fruit juices were thus shown to pose a greater erosive threat to these restorative materials than Coca-Cola. The findings for these drinks are similar for both enamel and dentine [21]. The influence of different dietary solvents (0.02 M citric acid, 50% ethanol–water solution, heptane, distilled water as control) on shear punch strength was determined. Results showed a lower strength for the nanofilled and ormocer composites than for the minifilled composite, but higher values than those achieved for the compomer and the highly viscous glass-ionomer cement [22]. Another investigation measured the effect of pH on the microhardness of a resin composite (Esthet-X, Dentsply DeTrey, Konstanz, Germany), a compomer (Dyract Extra, Dentsply DeTrey, Konstanz, Germany) and a giomer (Beautiful, Shofu, Kyoto, Japan). Results showed a material dependency: the compomer and giomer materials were more affected by acids than the composite material that was evaluated [23].

Regarding these investigations, the following conclusion can be made: Under acidic conditions all dental restorative materials show a degradation over time (surface roughness, decrease of surface hardness, substance loss). However, it seems that ceramic and composite materials show a good durability.

Treatment Strategies

Initial restorative treatments should be conservative, using adhesive materials [24]. Modern therapeutic concepts determine that minimal amounts of healthy tooth substance should be sacrificed. Reconstructive restorative treatments should be adapted to the tooth and not vice versa. However, when teeth wear, the alveolar bone and the associated tissues adapt to some degree to the change with alveolar compensation [25]. Despite losing crown height, teeth maintain their occlusal contact and this may lead to problems for their reconstruction because there is not enough space for the restorative material. To prevent an invasive, full mouth rehabilitation, it can be convenient to gain interocclusal space with orthodontic measures, especially if mainly groups of teeth (e.g. all teeth in the anterior region) are involved in erosive tooth wear. The orthodontic treatment can be achieved with fixed or removable appliances, such as the Dahl appliance [25]. Following orthodontic treatment, the eroded teeth can then be reconstructed [26]. Prior to the most recent decade, the severely eroded dentition could only be rehabilitated by the provision of extensive crown and bridge work, or in more severe cases, by means of removable overdentures [27–29]. As a result of the improvements in composite restorative materials and in adhesive techniques, it has become possible to rehabilitate eroded dentitions in a less-invasive manner. In recent years, the wear resistance of posterior composite fillings has been enhanced [8]. Therefore, the use of modern direct restorative materials can provide excellent longevity, even in load-bearing situations [11, 12]. Several case reports demonstrate the successful rehabilitation of (erosive) worn dentitions using adhesive techniques [30–33].

The restorative treatment plan should be adapted to the degree of tooth substance loss (e.g. loss of vertical dimension), as is mentioned above.

It should be kept in mind that erosive tooth wear is a multifactorial condition and in many cases it is not possible to determine and eliminate all etiological parameters. In such cases, the long-term success of the rehabilitation may be compromised.

Loss of Vertical Dimension <0.5 mm: Sealing or
Direct Composite Restoration

Treatment of erosive tooth wear should be performed at an early stage in order to prevent the development of functional and aesthetic problems. The most minimally invasive measure is the sealing of the tooth surface. In a study [34], Seal and Protect (Dentsply DeTrey, Konstanz, Germany) and Optibond Solo (Kerr, West Collins, Orange, Calif., USA) were each applied in vitro and in vivo. It was concluded that both products protected the teeth and the technique could be used clinically for patients. Another in vitro study examined the protective effect of adhesive systems on dentine after acid exposure and brushing abrasion in a cycling model. Twelve dentine samples each were pretreated with K-106 experimental varnish (Dentsply DeTrey, Konstanz, Germany), Prime & Bond 2.1 (Dentsply DeTrey), Syntac Classic with Heliobond (Vivadent, Schaan, Liechtenstein), Gluma Desensitizer (Heraeus Kulzer, Dormagen, Germany). Another twelve slabs served as the untreated control group. Each test sample was subjected 120 times to the following procedures: 5 min of demineralization (Sprite light), 1 h of storage in artificial saliva, brushing

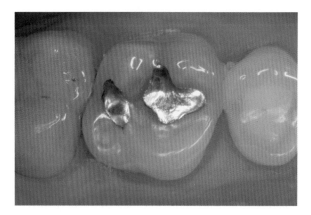

Fig. 1. Occlusal erosion with involvement of dentine. The edges of amalgam restoration are rising above the level of adjacent tooth surfaces.

abrasion (100 brush strokes) in an automatic brushing machine. Surface substance loss was measured by laser profilometry. It was concluded that adhesive systems can protect dentine from erosive tooth wear for a limited period of time [35]. Azzopardi et al. [36] investigated, in an in situ study, the surface effects of erosion and abrasion on dentine with and without a protective layer (Seal and Protect, Optibond Solo). Dentine sections were attached to an appliance and worn 8 h per day for 20 consecutive days. Every day the slabs were immersed in citric acid for 24 min. The effects of the acid exposure and the mechanical influence of the soft tissues, especially the tongue, on tooth surface substance loss were measured using four assessment techniques. Results showed that sealing materials remained in place despite a vigorous wear regime and therefore protected the tooth surface. The authors concluded that applying a dentine bonding agent to exposed dentine in patients with erosive tooth wear is a practical measure which prevents further damage. Clinical experiences show an obvious decrease of hypersensitivity of erosive damaged teeth after sealing. However, the sealing procedures have to be repeated periodically [37].

Occlusal erosions typically show grooves on occlusal aspects and edges of restorations are proud of the level of adjacent tooth surfaces. These grooves demonstrate a prolonged time of a depressed pH value after an acid attack [unpubl. obs.], which will lead to further progression of the erosive process at this site. In such cases, minimally invasive composite fillings are able to protect the affected region (figs. 1, 2). Conventional glass-ionomer cements are not recommended as permanent restorations because of their disintegration in acidic conditions [38].

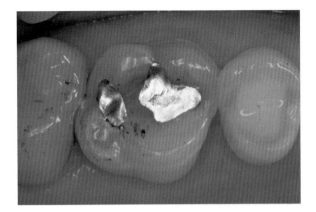

Fig. 2. The grooves of the molar were filled with composite after the cause (gastroesophageal reflux) was eliminated. The control of the occlusion is important to prevent early contact on the restoration (same case as fig. 1).

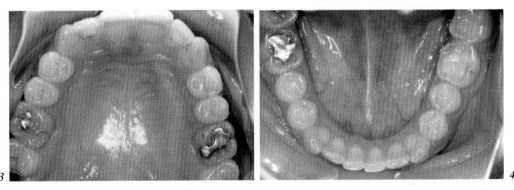

3 4

Figs. 3, 4. Occlusal and palatal erosion with involvement of dentine. Some restorations have been lost. The cause for the destruction was a history of previous bulimia. 1–1.5 mm of occlusal vertical dimension was lost. Direct composite restorations almost without preparation were planned.

Loss of Vertical Dimension <2 mm: Direct Reconstruction with Composite Materials

As long as there is only a loss of 1–2 mm of interocclusal space, the teeth can be reconstructed directly with composite materials. Patients tolerate such a small increase in the vertical dimension usually without any problem. Teeth are rebuilt 'freehand' according to their original anatomy (figs. 3–6). This

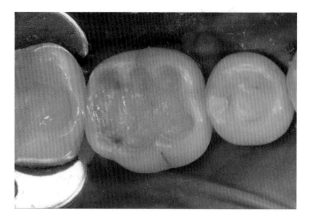

Fig. 5. Details of teeth 45 and 46 after removing the old restoration and after abrading the enamel and the dentine (same case as figs. 3, 4).

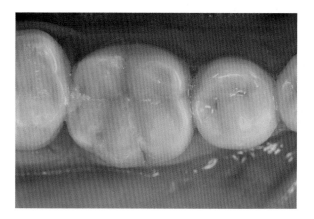

Fig. 6. Teeth 45 and 46 rebuilt with a direct composite restoration. Altogether, the vertical dimension was raised about 1.5 mm, which the patient tolerated without any difficulty (same teeth as fig. 5).

restorative measure can also be used for the reconstruction of localized facial or palatal surface defects (figs. 7, 8).

The advantage of direct composite restorations is that they are adaptable to the defect and repair is straightforward. The situation is more problematic if the occlusal and vestibular erosions merge, the original tooth shape becomes

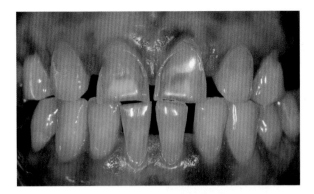

Fig. 7. Severe facial erosive defects with involvement of dentine on the central incisors (lemonslices under the lip).

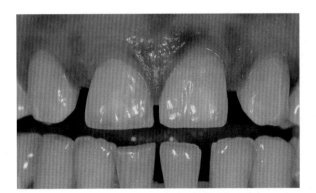

Fig. 8. Direct reconstruction with composite of teeth 11 and 21 (same case as fig. 7).

hardly recognizable and the loss of vertical dimension tends to be greater than 2 mm.

Loss of Vertical Dimension >2 mm: Rehabilitation with Indirect Ceramic Veneers and Overlays

In general, less-invasive reconstruction procedures such as direct adhesive methods are preferable to indirect methods. However, if the upper front teeth

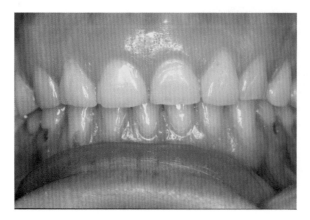

Fig. 9. Facial view of a patient with advanced erosive tooth wear. The incisal edges are abraded and the facial tooth surfaces show erosive defects (bulimic anorexia as a teenager).

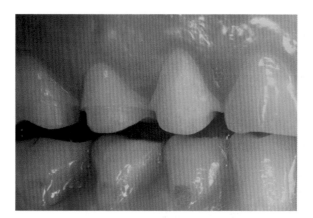

Fig. 10. Lateral view of the preparations of the upper right jaw. Expanding the preparation to that of a veneer preparation, including the facial erosive defect of tooth 14 (same patient as fig. 9).

are severely eroded and need to be reconstructed, porcelain veneers may sometimes be applied. If the defects (on posterior teeth) show an extension over two or more tooth surfaces and the vertical tooth substance loss is greater than 2 mm, then reconstruction with full ceramic overlays is convenient (figs. 9–12).

This treatment method demonstrates that aesthetic yet conservative reconstructions are possible with all-ceramic restorations. However, such treatment is expensive. Therefore, it is important to combine active treatment with preventive measures and recall at regular intervals to ensure the long-term success.

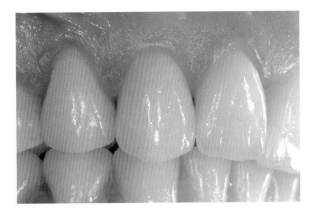

Fig. 11. Detailed view of the inserted ceramic veneers of teeth 12, 13 and 14 (same case as figs. 9, 10).

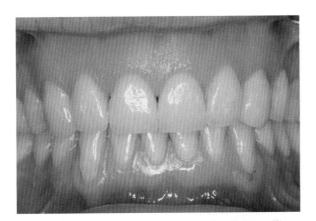

Fig. 12. Front view of the finished reconstructions: The upper incisors were reconstructed with 4 porcelain veneers, the canines with full ceramic crowns. The vertical dimension was increased in order to provide at least 1.5 mm thickness of the ceramic reconstructions (same case as figs. 9–11).

*Loss of Vertical Dimension >4 mm: Rehabilitation with
Indirect Ceramic Restorations*

In patients with severe tooth surface loss on more than two surfaces per tooth and extended loss of vertical dimension, a complex reconstruction with

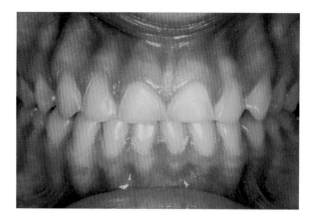

Fig. 13. Facial view of advanced dentinal erosions. Also the lower incisors have a clearly eroded silky lucent surface. Patient with a history of previous anorexia nervosa and with unfavorable (acidic) nutrition.

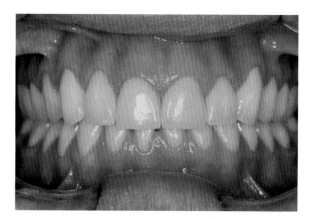

Fig. 14. Completed restoration of the upper and lower arches with full ceramic crowns and veneers on the lower incisors. The vertical dimension had to be increased for 4 mm in the anterior region. This increase was accomplished and tested step-by-step by means of provisional crowns. The patient did not have any problems adapting to the new vertical dimension and the treatment was therefore accomplished successfully (same case as fig. 13).

indirect restorations (ceramic crowns, bridges) is often inevitable. This measure should be restricted to very advanced erosion cases (figs. 13, 14). As in other patients with erosive tooth wear adequate preventive measures and recall intervals must be executed.

Acknowledgement

The authors thank Dr. Nicolas Widmer for providing some of the clinical pictures used in this chapter.

References

1   Amaechi BT, Higham SM: Dental erosion: possible approaches to prevention and control. J Dent 2005;33:243–252.
2   Vieira A, Ruben JL, Huysmans MC: Effect of titanium tetrafluoride, amine fluoride and fluoride varnish on enamel erosion in vitro. Caries Res 2005;39:371–379.
3   Lambrechts P, Van Meerbeek B, Perdigao J, Gladys S, Braem M, Vanherle G: Restorative therapy for erosive lesions. Eur J Oral Sci 1996;104:229–240.
4   Tay FR, Pashley DH: Resin bonding to cervical sclerotic dentin: a review. J Dent 2004;32:173–196.
5   Ogata M, Okuda M, Nakajima M, Pereira PN, Sano H, Tagami J: Influence of the direction of tubules on bond strength to dentin. Oper Dent 2001;26:27–35.
6   Ogata M, Harada N, Yamaguchi S, Nakajima M, Pereira PN, Tagami J: Effects of different burrs on dentin bond strengths of self-etching primer bonding systems. Oper Dent 2001;26: 375–382.
7   Van Dijken JW: Durability of three simplified adhesive systems in class V non-carious cervical dentin lesions. Am J Dent 2004;17:27–32.
8   Soderholm KJ, Richards ND: Wear resistance of composites: a solved problem? Gen Dent 1998;46:256–263.
9   Matis BA, Cochran M, Carlson T: Longevity of glass-ionomer restorative materials: results of a 10-year evaluation. Quintessence Int 1996;27:373–382.
10 Van Meerbeek B, Peumans M, Gladys S, Braem M, Lambrechts P, Vanherle G: Three-year clinical effectiveness of four total-etch dentinal adhesive systems in cervical lesions. Quintessence Int 1996;27:775–784.
11 Gaengler P, Hoyer I, Montag R: Clinical evaluation of posterior composite restorations: the 10-year report. J Adhes Dent 2001;3:185–194.
12 Manhart J, Garcia-Godoy F, Hickel R: Direct posterior restorations: clinical results and new developments. Dent Clin North Am 2002;46:303–339.
13 Nomoto R, McCabe JF: A simple acid erosion test for dental water-based cements. Dent Mater 2001;17:53–59.
14 Knobloch LA, Kerby RE, McMillen K, Clelland N: Solubility and sorption of resin-based luting cements. Oper Dent 2000;25:434–440.
15 Al-Hiyasat AS, Saunders WP, Sharkey SW, Smith GM: The effect of a carbonated beverage on the wear of human enamel and dental ceramics. J Prosthodont 1998;7:2–12.
16 Yap AUJ, Tan SHL, Wee SSC, Lee CW, Lim ELC, Zeng KY: Chemical degradation of composite restoratives. J Oral Rehabil 2001;28:1015–1021.
17 Shabanian M, Richards LC: In vitro wear rates of materials under different loads and varying pH. J Prosthet Dent 2002;87:650–656.
18 Turssi CP, Hara AT, Serra MC, Rodrigues AL Jr: Effect of storage media upon the surface micromorphology of resin-based restorative materials. J Oral Rehabil 2002;29:864–871.
19 Tsuchiya S, Nikaido T, Sonoda H, Foxton RM, Tagami J: Ultrastructure of the dentin-adhesive interface after acid-base challenge. J Adhes Dent 2004;6:183–190.
20 Gomec Y, Dorter C, Ersev H, Guray Efes B, Yildiz E: Effects of dietary acids on surface microhardness of various tooth-colored restoratives. Dent Mater J 2004;23:429–435.
21 Aliping-McKenzie M, Linden RWA, Nicholson JW: The effect of Coca-Cola and fruit juices on the surface hardness of glass-ionomers and 'compomers'. J Oral Rehabil 2004;31:1046–1052.
22 Yap AU, Lim LY, Yang TY, Ali A, Chung SM: Influence of dietary solvents on strength of nanofill and ormocer composites. Oper Dent 2005;30:129–133.

23 Mohamed-Tahir MA, Tan HY, Woo AA, Yap AU: Effects of pH on the microhardness of resin-based restorative materials. Oper Dent 2005;30:661–666.

24 Yip KH, Smales RJ, Kaidonis JA: The diagnosis and control of extrinsic acid erosion of tooth substance. Quintessence Int 2002;33:516–520.

25 Dahl BL, Krogstad O: The effect of partial bite raising splint on the occlusal face height. An X-ray cephalometric study in human adults. Acta Odontol Scand 1982;40:17–24.

26 Bartlett DW: The role of erosion in tooth wear: aetiology, prevention and management. Int Dent J 2005;4:277–284.

27 Hugo B: Orale Rehabilitation einer Erosionssituation. Schweiz Monatsschr Zahnmed 1991;101: 1155–1162.

28 Ganddini MR, Al-Mardini M, Graser GN, Almong D: Maxillary and mandibular overlay removable partial dentures for the restoration of worn teeth. J Prosthet Dent 2004;91:210–214.

29 Kavoura V, Kourtis SG, Zoidis P, Andritsakis DP, Doukoudakis A: Full-mouth rehabilitation of a patient with bulimia nervosa: a case report. Quintessence Int 2005;36:501–510.

30 Hastings JH: Conservative restoration of function and aesthetics in a bulimic patient: a case report. Pract Periodontics Aesthet Dent 1996;8:729–736.

31 Tepper SA, Schmidlin PR: Technik der direkten Bisshöhenrekonstruktion mit Komposit und einer Schiene als Formhilfe. Schweiz Monatsschr Zahnmed 2005;115:35–42.

32 Aziz K, Ziebert AJ, Cobb D: Restoring erosion associated with gastroesophageal reflux using direct resins: case report. Oper Dent 2005;30:395–401.

33 Bartlett DW: Three patient reports illustrating the use of dentine adhesives to cement crowns to severely worn teeth. Int J Prosthodont 2005;18:214–218.

34 Azzopardi A, Bartlett DW, Watson TF, Sherriff M: The measurement and prevention of erosion and abrasion. J Dent 2001;29:393–400.

35 Schneider F, Hellwig E, Attin T: Einfluss von Säurewirkung und Bürstabrasion auf den Dentinschutz durch Adhäsivsysteme. Dtsch Zahnarztl Z 2002;57:302–306.

36 Azzopardi A, Bartlett DW, Watson TF, Sherriff M: The surface effects of erosion and abrasion on dentine with and without a protective layer. Br Dent J 2004;196:351–354.

37 Lussi A, Jaeggi T, Schaffner M: Prevention and minimally invasive treatment of erosions. Oral Health Prev Dent 2004;2:321–325.

38 Yip HK, Lam WTC, Smales RJ: Fluoride release, weight loss and erosive wear of modern aesthetic restoratives. Br Dent J 1999;187:265–270.

Prof. Dr. Thomas Jaeggi
Department of Preventive, Restorative and Pediatric Dentistry
School of Dental Medicine
University of Bern
Freiburgstrasse 7
CH–3010 Bern (Switzerland)

Subject Index

progression rate assessment 40, 41
prospects 41
Distribution, erosive tooth wear 58–63, 95, 96

Eating disorders, *see* Anorexia nervosa; Bulimia nervosa
Ecstasy, erosive tooth wear risks 103, 104
EDTA, mouthwash content and erosive tooth wear risks 113
Electron microscopy, *see* Analytical transmission electron microscopy; Scanning electron microscopy
Electron probe microanalysis, element analysis of solid samples 165, 166
Enamel
    beverage adhesiveness and displacement effects on erosion 84
    chemical analysis 158, 159
    chemical composition 67, 68, 158
    mineral content in deciduous teeth 21
    softening 21, 94
    ultrasonic measurement of thickness 166
Endodontics, dentine hypersensitivity management 185
Erosion
    abrasion interactions 23
    attrition interactions 22, 23
    definition and etiology 9–11, 18, 21, 22
Exercise
    erosive tooth wear risks 102
    gastroesophageal reflux risks 125

Fasting, erosive tooth wear risks 103
Fluorapatite
    acid interactions 72
    tooth composition 67
Fluoride
    beverage supplementation 80
    dentine hypersensitivity management 181, 182
    erosion protection 80, 84, 94, 194, 196

Gastroesophageal reflux
    children 146, 147
    diagnosis and evaluation 124, 126, 127
    erosive tooth wear

association with specific symptoms 124
dental evidence for association 128, 129
medical evidence for association 127, 128
esophagus anatomy and physiology 120, 121
etiology 119, 120
risk factors
    alcohol 125
    diet 125
    exercise 125
    obesity 126
    posture 125
symptoms of gastroesophageal reflux disease 121–123
treatment 127

Herbal tea, erosive tooth wear risks 81, 102, 103, 192
Hunter-gatherers, tooth wear 12, 13
Hydrochloric acid tablets, erosive tooth wear risks 117
Hydroxyapatite
    acid interactions 72
    tooth composition 67

Incidence, erosive tooth wear 60–63
Iodine permeability test (IPT), principles 158
Iontophoresis, dentine hypersensitivity management 184, 185

Knoop diamond, surface hardness measurement 155, 156

Laser therapy, dentine hypersensitivity management 184

Microhardness, measurements 155, 156
Microradiography
    applications 160, 161
    longitudinal microradiography 161
    principles 159, 160
    transverse microradiography 160, 161